PURE TAOISM

by

the Barefoot Doctor

GETTING YOUR SOUL TO BLOOM

First published 2008

New edition published by Wayward Publications Ltd © (2017) Edinburgh

www.waywardpublications.com

Cover design Spanky Pymm

British Library Cataloguing-in-Publication Data

ISBN 978-1-912062-81-2 in epub format

ISBN 978-1-912062-82-9 in mobi format

ISBN 978-1-912062-83-6 in azw3 format

ISBN 978-1-912062-84-3 in pdf format

ISBN 978-1-912062-85-0 in print

Dedicated entirely to you

PURE fact

You are here and you are powerful.

And you block that.

You're blocking it as you read this.

That's OK and there are consequences.

One of these consequences is that you experience yourself as less than you are.

This leads you to experience life as less than it is.

That's OK too.

No one said you were obliged to get the full deal.

Meanwhile, you have this book in your hand and if you want more now, read on.

PURE elitism

This book is not a light read.

This book is not for lazy minds.

This book is not for those who like to be told what to do and how to live.

This book is not for those who think reading a book can change their lives.

This book is not for mugs, or those who believe themselves to be victims of circumstance.

This book is for those who have the courage to know what's what and not be fooled by the con of the modern world and all its false prophets.

This book is for those who know that only they can change their lives because it is only they who created their lives as they are in the first place, and for those who know that a book like this can be invaluable to their progress now.

This book is for those who are self-determining.

This book is for warriors.

This book is for you.

PURE struggle

Daily life – hard work sometimes, isn't it?

Confusing, irritating, frustrating, frightening, overwhelming and demanding, sometimes, isn't it?

Sometimes you want to get off.

Sometimes you're so scared you want to die.

Sometimes you're so torn with self-doubt you want to remove your own brain.

Sometimes you're so overloaded you want to run away – but where to?

You know that won't change anything.

You wish you could stop struggling with yourself.

You wish you could be more relaxed.

You wish you could be more of a master about it – be more cool more of the time.

But what if, instead of trying to change it, you stopped trying to change it?

What if you settled into it as it is, and accepted it – all the pain, all the strife, all the struggle, all the fear and all your apparent ineptness at managing it all with equanimity?

And what if you discovered, to your amazement, that by doing so, rather than congeal and transform into a potato-head, you actually attained the mastery that was eluding you?

Well, it could happen.

And here's how you'd do it.

PURE circles

That's what I'll be talking in. The universe is circular. There are no straight lines in existence, only the appearance of them. Extend any straight line into infinity and you will realize it's actually a section of a curve.

The information here derives from my interpretation of Taoism, an ancient Chinese system of life-management skills, all based on life being a circular affair.

Though in essence this information is so simple it could be succinctly presented on a single page, to achieve a sufficient understanding of the various factors involved to reach that simplicity requires a book's worth of space. And here we are.

If I could start at the beginning and work through progressively and systematically to the end in a straight line, I would, but there is no beginning, there is no end and there is no line – just a circular continuum of information-phases into which you could cut at any point and start from there, as in fact you're about to do now, if you are still reading.

PURE pretense

You're pretending. I'm pretending. We're all pretending here. We're all in disguise.

You look one way but you feel another. You project an air of confidence, as best you can, yet you are feeling scared and insecure.

You kid yourself you have it all under control in there but inside your mind is racing like a trapped monkey scampering frantically in a cage.

You act all grown-up and responsible but within you are a playful child.

You like to think butter wouldn't melt in your mouth but you're carrying enough guilt to build a house with (which is precisely what you've done inside yourself).

You walk proud, yet inside you feel ashamed.

You smile bravely, yet inside you are quivering with sadness and fear.

You feign disinterest, yet inside you are yearning.

It's all fake – mask upon mask upon mask.

You're doing it.

I'm doing it.

We're all doing it.

And it's all right. This is how we play the game of life with ourselves and each other.

Whatever you're showing hides a whole realm within of the exact opposite. And that realm hides another, the exact opposite to it, and so on. Layer upon layer of perspective after perspective.

However, behind all the masks and beneath all the layers, naked, beyond disguise, is the pure you. And that pure you is what some might call the Tao; others, God; others still, their higher self. But whatever you call it, it's ineffable and mysterious, defying definition. However, whether you attempt in vain to define or formalize it in any way or not, whether your intellect gels with it as a notion or not, you know it – you've touched it and it's touched you throughout your time here in the dream of life. It's what's been informing you, animating you and powering you on, every step of the way, from before the time you can consciously remember. It is you.

When you reach yourself in the fullness of your divine purity, the pretense falls away. It doesn't stop – the charade goes on – but you see straight through it, as if gazing through a phantasm. You still play. You still pretend – to yourself and to others – but you know you're doing it. And knowing you're doing it, that

13

which knows is your pure self, so the knowing becomes a device to be (with) your pure self. And the more you are (with) your pure self, the less the charade confuses you or obfuscates the process of manifesting what you want. Seeing through the pretense to who you really are, to what you are really feeling, to what you are really wanting, affords you simultaneous insight into who others really are, what they're really feeling and what they're really wanting.

And you know what that is?

Love.

That's what we are, what drives us on and what we want: love, the Tao, the juice of life, chi, the composite of absolute harmony, limitless power and infinite consciousness we all thrive on, but deny ourselves on account of getting distracted by the charade. Love comes in many forms – in fact, as many forms as there are. Everything is love made into a shape. The more expression love has in a form, the more beautiful that form becomes, whether mineral, plant, animal or human.

Love is purity. Purity is love. And words are words.

However, by following a few simple procedures, profound transformation of reality can be effected with hardly the lift of a finger and it is these simple procedures, along with clear explanations and instructions, which comprise the gift included between these pages for your existential and sensual delectation

14

and delight, along with some profound shifting for the better in all aspects of your existence.

PURE you

Beyond the everyday and the relative lies the realm of the absolute. Entry to this realm beyond reality – hyper-reality or hyperspace – grants access to personal powers beyond your everyday imagination, the sort of personal power associated with masters, one of the more exciting of which is being able to effect actual shifts in your relationships with others (the sum total of which comprises the structure of your personal world) and hence alter your external reality simply by intending it, and by doing so be able to actualize all your heart's true desires without strain, stress or any other unnecessary self-imposed enjoyment-blocking device, and so realize your full potential as a divine being in human form this very lifetime.

To enter hyper-reality, all that's required is that you be pure – it's easier for a camel to pass through the eye of a needle than for an impure person to pass into hyper-reality. Being pure, however, contrary to common misconception, has nothing to do with reducing the levels of toxicity in the food you eat, the water you drink, the air you breathe or the products you use, nor has it to do with whether you abstain from eating red meat or dairy, drinking alcohol, coffee or tea, or indulging in drugs, stimulants or chemicals of any kind.

Being pure has nothing to do with whether your mind loses itself in sexual fantasy, no matter how seemingly odd, twisted or perverted, nor with whether you ever catch yourself thinking nasty thoughts about others.

Neither does being pure mean never telling a lie, never indulging in malicious gossip, or only allowing good to spout forth from your lips.

Nor does being pure mean never engaging in masturbation or sex with others, even others that prevailing morals say you shouldn't be having sex with.

Being pure simply means being purely you – pure you – complete with all your imperfections, bad habits, quirks, ticks, vanities, conceits, deceits, obfuscations, miscellaneous murky odd bits and various skewed character aspects, as well as, of course, all your countless fine and noble qualities.

Only in this state of knowing, accepting and owning all of yourself, the dark as well as the light, can you be purely you and only by being purely you can you enter hyper-reality – the state of being in heaven-on-earth and the powers of the gods and Golden Immortals it confers on you.

This book is entirely about you, about you being you, knowing you, accepting you, owning you – the pure you – and thereby about you taking full command of yourself and your reality, as opposed to vice versa.

PURE acceptance

Exactly like everyone else on this planet, you are capable of and have the potential for the entire gamut of human thoughts, words and actions, from the loftiest to the lowliest, from the clearest to the most distorted, from the most constructive to the most destructive. This is true in any given moment; this present one, for instance.

Accepting this potential encompassing both extremes in yourself is prerequisite for growing fully into yourself, which is impossible as long as you're in denial of various aspects, whether the good or the bad, the healthy or unhealthy, the wise or the downright stupid. You cannot possibly hope to realize your full potential if you're in denial of one half of it.

If you split off the unhealthy parts, you cannot help also splitting off the healthy parts they were joined onto, until you own nothing of yourself and are merely a hollow shell living a pointless charade to yourself and others.

Owning your potential for harm does not encourage you to do more harm. Denying it and pushing it underground will make it rebel and cause you to act compulsively and harmfully.

19

Bringing it shuddering into the light of day and shining the light of awareness on it causes it to evaporate and leaves very little nasty after-smell. Remaining in denial of it and letting it fester, on the other hand, creates an unpleasant odor, which though only discernable on the subtle level, will nonetheless keep the sensitive-nosed emissaries of opportunity and good fortune away from you.

So, step one of becoming pure comprises owning up to the dark aspects of yourself, as well as to the bright, shining ones.

To assist yourself here, you might wish to take a moment to list whatever you secretly find disgusting about yourself.

Then, lest you remain fixated on the negative, make a list of everything you admire about yourself – everything you approve of about yourself – everything you love yourself for.

Then look at the two lists comprising all your aspects and realize they only reflect one level of your existence, which after all is essentially subjective, relative and hence illusory anyway – just a matter of opinion, and opinions are as consistent and meaningful as the breeze. You are not this. You are neither the disgusting nor the admirable and you are both, and as soon as you acknowledge, accept and integrate the two, they cancel each other out anyway, leaving you with who you really are – pure you, the Tao. That's how big this is. No limits.

PURE insanity

There can hardly be anything more mad and unlikely than human society – what we usually mean when we refer to the world. It is purely insane.

The world is apparently overcrowded now in all respects and we no longer know how we're going to sustain ourselves. Tensions are exponentially growing individually, socially, economically, ecologically, politically, militarily and quasi-militarily.

We have never faced a greater risk to our everyday survival.

We know even the use of the word 'everyday' is a palliative to soothe frightened minds, for we're aware that what we conceive of as the everyday could be drastically upended by any number of factors at any moment.

Yet amidst this insanity lies great sanity, both collectively and individually.

Each of us has a direct line through to it.

Each of us has the capacity to access it and trigger its spread for the benefit of all of us.

The more of us that do this, the greater the chance we have of promoting survival and evolution and this is the only chance we've got.

Whether we take advantage of this capacity or choose to remain in the deluded, insane state, is entirely up to us.

If your choice is to create the possibility of participating in a world promoting survival and evolution, in which you also manifest everything you desire to make your life go with that swing that would make you feel like the queen or king, this book is here to provide one way to implement that choice with optimum effect.

As I say, all the information it contains originates from Taoism, which in turn originates from ancient China – as far as we know. Some believe it originated in outer space.

Taoism is merely a more or less lazy title for an ancient system of training yourself in a set of ingeniously devised, universally pertinent, life-management skills, working mostly with the mind but also through the body in quite a physical sense – it's a psychophysical system, in other words.

This book is intended as a feasible vehicle through which to pass on the crucial aspects of the training for your potential benefit, the extent of which depends entirely on the degree to which you actually practice what you read here (and there is no obligation on your part), as well as which it provides the possibility that through these words, I might entertain and inspire you as you wend your way to work of a morning, or sit on the toilet, or lie in bed, or whatever. For though, of course, I exhort you with all my heart to fully immerse yourself in it and let it work its magic without hindrance, I would say whether you practice the techniques or action the philosophical stances I suggest, and thereby implement a transformation in your life or not, providing you like reading non-fiction, you won't necessarily have wasted your money or time, as this book's probably as good as any other, providing you're in the mood, and I dare say the very act of allowing the thoughts it inspires to roll round your mind while reading it will have a talismanic effect in the sense of transforming the context of your reality and thereby the content. But if you actually adopt what's in the book and use it on a daily basis, both the qualitative and quantitative difference it could make to your reality, in all respects, could be profound and huge.

PURE form

Your body, as well as being the vehicle through which you express yourself and conduct your interactions in the world, is also the arena in which you feel the Tao and so touch perfection, while enjoying the sensual excitement of being alive. Whether you find yourself in quiet spiritual contemplation or in the thrilling midst of the external stimulation-driven hubbub – it all goes on inside your body.

When you allow yourself to be body-centered with your awareness, rather than rational-mind-centered, your intuition comes to the fore and guides you every step of the way. Following this intuition – or, literally, tuition from within – is how you navigate hyper-reality and, by extension, regular workaday reality too.

When your awareness is rational-mind-centered, the tendency is to keep repeating familiar patterns because that's all your rational mind really knows and while that works on one level to keep you regular in your activities, it prevents you being in the fullness of yourself and so diminishes whatever value you're gaining from being alive.

When your awareness is body-centered, your rational mind does fine on its own, working out everything required to keep the show on the road in a logistical sense, which is what you need it for. It will give you all the headlines you require for survival and won't actually need you interfering all the time to fulfil that function.

With this combination in place, with this relationship sorted, with the mental and physical, the spiritual and profane, the light and the dark in balance, you are fully you and hence pure. It's my sincere aim in writing this book to aid you to be fully pure, so that by the time you reach the last letter of the last word on the last page you will, if you have paid attention and done as suggested to some extent, touched a state of unshakeable yet fluid oneness with yourself, with the essence of the world around you and with all who sail in her. And with the Tao informing it all. You will be living pure, as in fully authentic and fully yourself, and so fully energized and capable of achieving anything you set your mind to, easily, effortlessly, enjoyably and miraculously. From that point on, it'll be up to you, in terms of whether you adopt long-term any of the practices or philosophies so you can sustain this.

'I knew all that anyway,' you'll say. And that'll be fine because you do.

PURE mess

Being purely yourself will in no way preclude you from making a proper mess of it at times, but it will be pure mess. Plus there must be an element of mess in every life, to serve as a viable contrast to the pure harmony you'll be experiencing progressively more of the time by being purely you, so it might as well be pure mess.

Indeed, by the time you get to the end of this book, you'll be staring pure mess straight in the eye and saying, 'Bring it on, buddy,' because you know that every piece of pure mess has a miracle of harmony and resolution hidden within its folds, awaiting your discovery.

It's all to do with good staging. The Tao loves theater, so it plays with tension and release. Mess engenders tension which then finds release as reality transforms itself into something more harmonious again. Without the mess, the miracle would get commonplace, thus depriving you of the thrill of existence and without that you're really wasting time.

Don't take the phases of tension and release, mess and miracle too seriously, however. Instead, relax and enjoy it. It's just theatre – all of it.

Do you believe that?

PURE belief

A prerequisite is that you have to believe. It doesn't matter what in. Belief is the key to hyper-reality. Believe me when I say that. You have to believe this is a book to read it.

You have to believe in the meaning you give the words or you can't make sense of them.

You have to believe you're here reading it or none of it makes any sense.

By believing you transform potential into the actual.

Believe in purity as the way to hyper-reality and it will be so.

Believe purity consists in being purely you and it will be so.

That's how reality organizes itself. It's not a one-way street. You shape reality as it's shaping you.

You shape it with belief – belief in the Tao, in the natural flow of things, in yourself, in the ineffable, in Sid The Barber of Commercial Road. It makes no difference how you try in vain to define it, all that matters is you believe.

Believing is a mode, a sensation of energy and intention for forward momentum arising in the belly and chest; a reaching in to reach out to the invisible conscious force informing and animating all of this.

Believing constitutes your commitment to the adventure of life. Without belief you're nothing – at best you're a shiny shell, at worst demented.

See what you want spread out before you in your imagination. Believe you can cause it all to come to pass. Feel it in your belly and chest. Hear yourself saying, 'I can do it,' and let that I-can-do-it resound throughout your person. It may only last a split second but in that instant you are believing, you are substantiated by that belief and that belief will draw you along your path towards the goal of total self-fulfilment and self–realization.

It's in a state of belief that all the real magic is effected. Ask any real magician, or better still, ask the Great Magician, the Tao.

PURE Tao

The Tao is just a word, a monosyllabic phonic outblurt, not much more than an uncouth grunt, alluding to something simply too huge to explain with words. It comprises the pre-atomic, primordial, supra-conscious, intelligent generative force of all existence, manifesting, informing and animating all its infinite aspects and manifestations – including you and me and all other sentient beings – not just here on the planet, but throughout time and space in all possible dimensions simultaneously.

As the sum total of all the ineffable intelligence of the universe and everyone in it, it stands to reason you can enter into a dialogue with it in a same-but-different way to the idea of praying in the conventional sense to any essentially divine entity. However, it differs from the traditional style of praying in that you don't look upwards towards a higher being, you look both inwards and all around you on the level, for that's where it's to be found at all times, without exception.

As an expression of the Tao, you are a divine being yourself.

Whenever you're tuned in sufficiently to feel the Tao within and around you, you are a channel of the divine – and as such, you have no need to delude yourself further about being less than it or any other entity (this isn't a size contest, in any case, and the entire universe can be found in an atom). From now on, you're on the level with it. The Tao is your friend – the best and ultimately only friend you have in the entire universe, so you have no need to feel afraid of it, subservient to it, reverent towards it, or in any way inferior to it. Safely assume that the Tao does not enjoy you indulging in such delusions of inequality and nothing will be gained thereby.

The Tao is often described as the Mother of all Existence, implying a soft, gentle, nurturing sensation on offer when you enter into dialogue with it, rather than something possibly harsh, male or authoritative. The Tao has authority only in the sense that it is the author of the storyline of existence, which it writes through each of us as we go along, hence the notion that we each create, or, more precisely, co-create, our own realities.

Relax and trust and you instantly create a reality you can relax into and trust. It's as simple and simplistic as that.

When you do that and so find you're in dialogue with the Tao, in hyper-reality, you are granted the power to trigger quantum events or so-called 'miracles' in your daily life. However, remember that dialogue is a two-way phenomenon and the art is to learn to listen and hear what the Tao is saying back to you. This it does via prompts and urges in your body and energy field, which you discern and translate into human-level thought, whereby you are drawn to either this or that, which you discern and translate into human thought. It is through hearing and following these messages that your deepest adventure unfolds.

The Tao also speaks to you through other people – which is obvious if you bear in mind that the Tao is informing everyone in your world, not just you, so will express itself via the actions and words of others, as well as directly through you.

Understanding what the Tao is telling you will not be achieved through the intellect or rational mind – the intellect merely deciphers and sorts the information for you. Understanding comes of itself through attaining pure thought as a result of following your intuition.

PURE thought

Pure thought, of which intuition is the envelope, has nothing to do with chastity of mind – it has nothing to do with the content of your thoughts whatsoever. Pure thought is all to do with how you think – context rather than content, in other words. And how you think is determined by where you think, as in which part of the brain you're choosing to use.

The habitual tendency is to use the forebrain exclusively. The prefrontal lobes are where the internal commentary and discussion about your life, or what you're perceiving as your life, goes on incessantly, distracting you from being the divine being you really are. You use this self-disguising device, in fact, to preclude you having to know yourself as divine, because once you know yourself as divine, with the power to effect miracles in daily life, you are responsible – you have to take active responsibility for your life. While you're fixated on the mental activity in the forebrain, you are able to indulge the illusion that you are not responsible for your life, but a victim of the world around you and therefore powerless.

However, if you train yourself to draw your mind backwards into the midbrain, in a real, tangible, psycho-spatial way, you instantly radically shift the very ground of your being and will start looking at the world with the (responsible and therefore empowered) eye of the Tao.

Spread out from pure reading mode for a moment and massage the roof of your mouth with the tip of your tongue in a clockwise circular motion approximately nine times. Now gently push your neck back. Somewhere in front of the vanguard of your forward thrust and behind the sensation just engendered in the roof of your mouth, is the central brain region. The ancient Taoists, who hailed from (ancient) China, referred to this region of the brain as the cavity (or cave) of original spirit. Anatomically it relates approximately to the pineal gland.

By training yourself to draw your awareness back to this point and to observe, bear witness to and experience reality from this point at all times, you go beyond reality in the midst of the everyday, to the realm of causation. So that as you attend to whatever you're doing, you have your feet firmly on the ground rooted in mundane reality, while simultaneously enjoying the universal thrill of being the Tao, the divine and are therefore with the power to shift external conditions as if by thought and intention alone. It's the best rush available, when you get it right. That just takes practice and the only thing in the way of that happening is you.

PURE resistance

Resistance to the new is a sign of strength – honor it. There will always be resistance to assimilating fresh information and putting it to good use, no matter how sound or resonant that information is. The degree of resistance will depend on how long it takes your mind to evaluate whether to allow the new in, or whether to resist it for fear of it unbalancing the established mix of beliefs and world-view. Because the information about to come to you, assuming you continue reading, requires daily practice in terms of developing various skills apropos how you use your mind, body and energy, it is natural for there to be resistance – both on initially reading the words and on adopting the content as part of a daily (or nightly, or both) regimen of self-regulation, self-healing and self-development.

Which is fine, as long as you find it useful. Honor resistance as a sign of strength. At the same time, however, also recognize that strength is often misplaced, which might well be the case should you find yourself resisting something that can cause your whole life to be transformed for the better to an immeasurable measure. You might also want to look at how you perhaps remain in the discomfort of not expressing yourself fully and therefore miss fulfilling your potential, because you've grown habituated to it and are afraid of attaining the genuine comfort of being fully yourself (which, remember, is nothing less than the Tao), in case you enjoy it too much – for then what would you have to moan about?

PURE wisdom

We like to suffer.

We do everything we can to avoid suffering.

We're crazy mixed-up beings.

There is no resolution to this.

Accepting the paradox without seeking resolution is pure wisdom.

However, we make this state and the inner peace it confers difficult for ourselves to attain because our meaning-craven minds feel a need to distract us by attempting in vain to resolve all paradoxes, as if that will then make life's meaning clear, when it was patently clear all along. And so we suffer. The only meaning life has is the meaning we ourselves give it, though if you're insightful and honest with yourself, you'll probably agree with me: namely that the bulk of the meaning you've given it so far is of it being an unfathomable experience providing you with an invaluable opportunity for as much enjoyment as you can possibly manage to accommodate without bursting, while you do all you can to shield yourself from pain as far as possible without making the story overly slushy. And if so, I say more power to you. To the furtherance of this you can ascribe the benefits of loving people and sharing times of reinforcing each other's sense of wellbeing and self-esteem via an infinite variety of mutual entrancement (or entertainment – literally, holding the space between you and the other), this act we're presumably engaging in now, for instance, of you entrancing me by playing your role as (potentially imaginary, from my point of view) reader, and me entrancing you by playing my role as writer. Which could also possibly be imaginary, to be fair – you never know, I may be just a computer-generated program or ghost writer – perhaps Barefoot left the building long ago – who can ever really tell, the way we manipulate reality these days?

And who knows, maybe you're not there either – you certainly won't be if I don't finish writing this book, at least not there reading this. But I will finish, of that you can be sure – in fact the proof lies in your hand in case you were doubting me, which in itself provides a poignant example of destiny being made manifest by intention and lots of key-tapping alone and being only really provable in retrospect. And of course, that could all just be…

PURE bullshit

I've said this already, but I will say it again.

Purity has nothing to do with the stuff you say, think or do, no matter the poisons you take in or put out.

Purity, however, has everything to do with doing everything you do with the fullness of your person, with the totality of your self, including all the dark and all the light, brought fully to bear on each and every moment through each and every thought, word and deed. When you're coming from the fullness of yourself, not in self-denial or self-deception about who you really are, the pureness of your self at the deepest level will shine through. So even when you're lying your tits off, if you're doing it with the fullness of self brought to bear on what we all know is a short-sighted but occasionally expedient strategy for managing relations with others, you are being pure – a pure bullshitter.

Of course, that could all be pure bullshit and probably is, whichever way you look at it.

As it happens, in case you were starting to wonder, no matter how much it may seem to the contrary just now, I'm not trying to confuse you – play with you, yes, but not at your expense – play with you as two friends play together, investigating reality and hyper-reality for the sheer hell (or heaven) of it. I'm not trying to confuse you, however. Perhaps I'm trying to tire our rational minds enough for us to suspend judgment here for long enough for us to delve together into the depths of our respective psyches, so that we might meet beyond the trance of the humdrum and beyond the level of preferences of right over wrong or vice versa in the realm of causation and thus produce, each in his own reality, a completely different and vastly improved and expanded set of conditions, but before we even attempt such feats of metaphysical acrobatics, it really is time we finally got off our misconceived, childish notions of what is pure.

What we may have thought of hitherto as pure is a totally unattainable state that could only exist in our imagination, in the realm of the ideal – and we all know that's only for babies. Forsooth, even St Francis of Assisi or the Buddha himself would have had the occasional lustful, deceitful, vicious or subversive thought in their all-but-pristine lifetimes. You can be as sure of that as you can be that without defecation, a person dies – not everything in this world can be sweet-smelling, however hard we try and mask the unpleasantness, in other words; so let us be real now.

Be yourself, in short, and you are pure: purely you, and that includes all your so-called impurities and bad habits. And the irony is that the more often you identify with the pure state within, the more pure you start being in your thought, word and deed, but not because you're forcing it and hence being impure in your purity – you're doing it by being pure in your impurity.

But how to be that? And what is it in the first place, this self of yours you have to be to be pure with? And what are the advantages of being so (according to me)?

PURE delight

When you are being fully 100 per cent you, with no consideration for the expectations of others, with no thought for whether you're being an idiot, with no care for the outcome, and with no fear of the consequences; and when this state has arisen, not from denial but from being fully in your skin, inhabiting all of yourself from head to toe and from front to back and back to front, from inside out and outside in, from above and from below, your breath flowing in and out freely without interruption (unless with need to hold it when swimming underwater without equipment, when passing through toxic regions or when someone has released foul gases in close proximity to your person), and when your heart is relaxed and beating to the rhythm of the world, permitting your innate human warmth and loving intelligence to flow to all parts within and around you, and when you can observe the entire show and unfolding of events from back in the midbrain region, rather than from up front in your eyeballs, you will find yourself in an undeniable state of pure delight. You are literally filled with light. Light comes from the sun. You and the sun are one – and do bear in mind, contrary to western religious conditioning, the sun is our local point of ineffable, inexplicable, presumably divine light. This does not mean the sun is a god. There's no mumbo jumbo like that involved. It means the sun is our nearest point in space through which the light of life expresses itself in reality – not in your imagination. And seeing as this world of ours and eventually everything in and on it, including the machinery and technology that are both saving and destroying us, originally all sprang forth from the sun, along with the consciousness driving it all, you could reckon yourself to be standing on fairly safe, reliable ground by going along with the idea that the drive for delight is an innate yearning to reconnect with the source of being and that by so doing you are connected to the source of being and when that happens you don't need alcohol or drugs to make you feel better, you just need to keep it all going like that and not trip yourself up by telling yourself the wrong story about what's going on.

PURE fiction

Reality, as you perceive it, is the result of a story you're telling yourself. Tell yourself a different story about it and reality changes. Don't ask me how that works. Ask a quantum physicist who experiments on the cutting edge. In any case, it doesn't matter how it works. Trying to figure out how things work does not bring enlightenment, the attainment of which is the subtext of this book – enlightenment, mastery of self and the material plane, call it what you will. Experimenting without knowing how, on the other hand, will lead to enlightenment, providing certain principles are adhered to. Then the mysteries of how things work will reveal themselves of themselves – at least that's how it worked for Einstein – and it will work well enough for you too.

These principles will be enumerated and explained in some depth as the pages unfold but for now, let's stay with an investigation into the story you're telling yourself. Do you believe the world is hostile, for instance? If so, that's the story you're telling yourself – you inhabit a hostile place. Your whole strategy for life will then be predicated on that premise, causing the signals you emit to invite hostility. This mechanism occurs to prove you right – life will always prove you right. That's one of its qualities.

However, if you believe the world is supportive, like a universe-sized mother whose only function is to sustain and nurture you and facilitate the occurrence of conditions that will make you perfectly happy, then that's the story you're telling yourself about it and the signals you unconsciously emit will convey that and invite support from the world in all your endeavors. Life will prove you right, in other words, and providing you don't then get in the way by, for example, telling yourself a duff story to counter it, on account of simultaneous innate feelings of shame or worthlessness inculcated from distorted parenting, perhaps somewhere around the same time as you originally wrote yourself the happy story, you will be perfectly happy... Look at the story you're telling yourself.

Implicit, here, is the option to tell yourself a totally different story at any time. Of course, this has to be done thoughtfully and at a time of great inner stillness, for to attempt such a profound passage of dialogue with yourself when the mind is distracted by the external effects of whatever story you're been telling yourself till now is all but impossible.

Hence the value of training yourself to meditate on some kind of regular basis.

That's right. Nothing comes for free. You have to do something for it. Your relationship with life is reciprocal. It's a two-way exchange.

Learn to still your raging thoughts and the Tao, your Tao, your Way, will afford you the ability to create whatever story you fancy and the effects will be profound, radical and far-reaching. But bear in mind that this, too, is a story. I'm telling you a story that life as you know it is a result of the story you're telling yourself about it. And if you buy this story from me and adopt it as your own, that's how it will be because that's the story you're telling yourself about it. There are no rules outside that. That's how plastic reality actually is – providing you believe that to be so. If not, we can't play. For playing this is, as I said before. I don't even know what the results will be for you and take no responsibility for them in any case. You must be the one to do that. You, on your own, on your own path and by your own responsibility – it's you who's creating all this, not me.

I'm busy creating my own version, even as I share it with you.

However, I do know you will undergo radical transformation if you do decide to play.

Whether that's a good thing or not, I don't know either, but good and bad are merely relative terms anyway. What looks good today can look equally bad tomorrow and vice versa – I'm assuming you're mature enough to have concluded that by now.

I'm assuming I am too.

We can never really tell till tested. But even the idea of being tested is just part of a story. In fact, I'm quite up for relinquishing that aspect of the story right now if you are.

An end to tests.

From now on, let's substitute tests for materializations along the way to us attaining our respective states of pure happiness.

PURE happiness

Bask in that for a moment – pure happiness – with no tests and nothing to prove. Imagine it, luxuriate in it. Don't fight it. Don't allow your mind to sully or besmirch it. Stay with it. Pure happiness. Not a smidgeon of unhappiness in the mix. Imagine it. Feel it. That's good. You just experienced pure happiness. Not many can make such a claim.

And the only reason it can't last is you can't let it. And you know why? Because you've told yourself a story that says you can't. Are you happy with that story so far?

Truthfully?

Yes, I know you can rationalize it – I do it all the time. Pure happiness cannot last because of all the suffering within and around. But what if you told yourself a story including pure happiness as your natural state, in which the only thing preventing it going on perpetually was your belief that the suffering had to stand in opposition to it? Imagine that you could accommodate the suffering along with the happiness and that the resulting force of pure happiness was so strong it transmuted all suffering in its path. Well, it is if you choose it to be, if you write it into the story.

If you notice something repetitive in my style of driving my message home – something repetitive in my style of driving my message home – this is entirely intentional. As I say, the gist of what I'm saying is so simple, the whole book could be written on one page. So I'm taking full advantage of the multiple-page format of books to drive home my point.

The simplest things need constant repetition to be effective in terms of transformation.

Repeat 81 times without hesitation, 'This is all just a story I'm telling myself.'

PURE consciousness

To perceive heaven and plug into the transformative power available to you in any single moment, your mind must be pure. It must be free of the noise coming off your forebrain, where the internal debate is constantly raging. You can't turn the debate off, but you can disengage from it, as previously stated, by gathering your consciousness into the center of your brain.

Drawing your consciousness back and gathering it in the center of your brain comprises one of the greatest tricks for transforming perception, and hence external reality, known to humankind. It is as old as the hills and provides the key to being fully in command of yourself and your experience of existence. So now expand beyond reading mode to experiential mode again and turn your head slowly and sensitively from side to side. As you do, tune into the sensation at the point of turn. A thumb's width above that in the direction of your crown, you'll feel your midbrain region, more or less equidistant between your ears. It's important to get a tangible sensation of the midbrain. Spend as much time as it takes, over a period of days if necessary, until you can tune into the physical sensation of the midbrain.

Once you know where it is physically, start using it as an eye. Literally start using it to gaze out at the world from, relegating your eyeballs themselves to playing the role of mere lens-covered openings in the front of the skull.

You'll instantly feel your experience of being here in your body, reading this, deepening. You'll feel yourself experiencing being here from deeper inside you.

This causes external reality to reflect that back at you by displaying its deeper aspects – the layers of life and consciousness occurring beneath the charade of the everyday, held in place by the trance of the humdrum.

If you're in a sensitive mood, you may feel the Tao caressing you. To help the sensation along, gently push your neck backwards a bit. Spend a few moments with your eyelids lowered almost all the way down, allowing just a slither of light in at the bottom to keep you awake, gazing from midbrain into the endless expanse of infinite inner space between and behind your eyes.

You'll notice at once that the usual tumult of noise issuing forth from the front of the brain, which is where all the internal chit-chat about how life is and should be, where the commentary on the storyline is, has gone amazingly quiet. You'll then be said to be experiencing pure consciousness. The tricky bit is keeping it up. Hence the value of repetitive practice, repetitive practice.

PURE simplicity

You can make life as complex as you like but that's all stuff of the mind – fodder for the internal debate. It all boils down to being here in the moment in your body, breathing in and out – all the rest is in your head. This is true without exception, no matter how vigorously your rational mind doth protest.

Furthermore, talking of what's in your head, the quality and tone of your breathing directly influence the quality and tone of your thoughts. When your breath is rough and uneven, your thoughts are crude and unbalanced. When your breath is smooth and even, your thoughts are refined and just.

Refine the breathing process and you refine your consciousness. Refine your consciousness and you refine the quality of your external conditions – like attracts like in a trans-dimensional sense. As above, so below; as within, so without. This is the cardinal rule of doing magic in your life. Attend to the inner and the outer attends to itself.

You labor under the illusion that the goal is to sort out what's in your head and thereby sort out what's going on in your life, whereas the goal is to simply be here, breathing in and out in such a peaceful way that the thoughts in your head sort themselves out without you getting involved, which causes external conditions to match that by sorting themselves out without you getting involved.

Draw your consciousness back into your midbrain and focus from there on the way you're breathing down below.

Relax your diaphragm and stop holding your breath.

By inhibiting your breath, you're inhibiting your whole life. Breath is life. One of the main things you notice about a dead person is that they're not breathing. Breath is life. Breathing in fills you with fresh life. Breathing out releases the stale, used-up life from your system, both physically and psycho-emotionally.

By holding tension in your diaphragm, thereby inhibiting the movement of breath coming in, you limit the amount of new life and hence opportunities and healthy growth possible in your reality in any one moment. By holding onto the breath instead of exhaling freely, you hold onto and absorb toxins both physically and psycho-emotionally, hence why holding your breath perpetuates a state of negativity (toxicity) in the mind, which then goes on to affect your physical and material states.

Expand beyond reading mode again and relax your thoracic cavity (chest and upper back).

Allow your belly to swell to accommodate the in-rushing air and then actively flatten it by pulling the muscles back towards the spine to push the air back out again, or rather vice versa.

Start by flattening the belly to expel the stale air. The more stale air you expel, the more fresh air the lungs will automatically take in on the inhalation.

This initially requires a modicum of effort in retraining the belly muscles to correspond with the breath, but with only a few days' practice you'll be doing it automatically a lot of the time, not because you think you should but because at an autonomic level you will have noticed that it feels way better and you will have naturally addicted yourself to it.

PURE addiction

Addiction, or homeostasis, is the force reality uses by which to organize itself into viable structures. There's nothing intrinsically wrong with it. It's what you addict or don't addict yourself to that counts. Addictiveness is a yin propensity. The yin urge is to habitually organize structures out of nothing by forming pre-atomic patterns and perpetuating them, in order to lend material reality substance, shape and duration. Yang force provides the thrust for change. Yin defends and organizes reality into something appearing static, yang represents dynamism. The friction between these two, as they lock in eternal struggle for homeodynamic balance, results in what we perceive as the constant war between the conservative and progressive forces both in society and in ourselves, without which things wouldn't stay in form long enough for material reality to exist on the one hand, or would congeal and implode on the other.

In your own life you need the one to feed the other, a balance you effect primarily by breathing freely in and out at a slow, steady tempo and making the in-breath, representing the yin,

57

of equal duration to the out-breath, representing the yang. It's that simple/simplistic, yet it is also utterly profound. When seeking balance in your life, it all begins with the breath. Once the breath is balanced, your body's intelligence automatically balances the amount of time required in any one moment, or phase, for resting versus activity.

Along with maintaining your consciousness in the center of your brain, letting yourself get addicted to breathing freely in and out at a slow, steady tempo and making the in-and out-breaths of equal duration is potentially extensively beneficial.

Some addictions are useful, others are not. This internally-produced combination drug I'm pushing you here is one of the useful ones.

The more you indulge it, the less you'll be inclined to indulge the useless or harmful ones.

And it's free.

Moreover, when your consciousness is gathered in the center of your brain, putting you instantly in command of your reality, you're at liberty to ascribe any quality you choose to both the breath coming in and the breath leaving. There are no rules in that respect. For instance, you can imbue the in-breath with the essence of courage, strength and vitality and grant the out-breath the power to carry away all your doubt, weakness and unhealthy resistance. You could breathe in life and breathe out death, or breathe in peace and breathe out stress, or breathe in love and breathe out fear. But you've got to be in the mood, or you miss the magic and it becomes boring. In that case, breathe in patience and sensitivity to subtlety and breathe out impatience and crudeness of mind. Then breathe in success and breathe out failure. Breathe in purity and breathe out impurity. Watching and enjoying yourself doing it from the center of your brain, the next thing you'll be wanting to take on board to milk the high is the correct positioning and alignment of the most important bit of physical structure about you: your spinal column.

PURE uplift

Imagine yourself in some sort of observation platform at the top of a skyscraper which hasn't been built properly and is leaning to the left, the right, the back or the front at such an angle it is placing severe strain on the foundations of the building. First, unless you are half-asleep, you'll be feeling fairly unsafe. Second, you'll be using energy to compensate for the tilt, in order to maintain some sort of upright stance. Third, with the tower leaning, your natural inclination will be to look down, thus instigating a downward magnetic pull of your person towards the ground.

Imagine how much safer you'd feel if the building righted itself. Imagine how much less energy you'd require to hold yourself upright, instead of fighting not to slip down the tilting floor, and how much brighter your outlook would be now your line of vision is straight outwards, encompassing the sky as well as the ground, as opposed to being fixated solely on the ground where all the shadows lurk.

Imagine that observation platform is situated in the center of your brain and the skyscraper supporting it is your spine.

Then return to real time and check your posture. (Mirrors are useful in this instance.) You'll probably find yourself inclining one way or another, or possibly two ways at once (forward and to the side, for instance). To afford that pure part of you bearing witness in the center of the brain the equilibrium it warrants, gently right the building by elongating your spine.

To do so, imagine someone gently raising the top of your skull by way of an invisible thread attached to your crown and feel the vertebrae separating to afford you more length. Assist this by pushing your neck back a bit.

Simultaneously attend to any sideways tilt.

With your skull sitting straight atop your newly elongated spine, you'll notice your outlook immediately brightens, your mind clears and your energy and spirits lift.

Keep breathing freely down below all the while.

PURE gravitas

Because there's nothing intrinsically heavy about being in hyper-reality – indeed, it comprises a state of supreme lightness – you need to be grounded and in touch with the telluric energy beneath your feet, in order to anchor the experience in the physical realm, moment-by-moment. You have to allow the energy of the ground to rush up through you, to empower you with the pre-atomic yin, substantive energy, which ironically you do by consciously transferring the weight of your head and upper parts downwards, allowing it to sink down below the level of the navel, thence to settle in your hips and legs. This will not make your belly, hips and legs fat, incidentally. On the contrary – it will increase circulation in those parts, thus making for slenderness and perky tone of muscle all round.

So as you sit, stand, or lie there with your consciousness gathered back in the center brain region, the breath flowing freely, slowly and smoothly down below and the spinal column lengthened to hold you upright and aligned, simultaneously allow your weight to sink below your navel and tune into the fact that the ground you're on is part of the surface of a planet spinning at 1000 mph on its axis, while orbiting the sun at 66,000 mph, thereby supplying and transmitting to anything resting on its surface an almost unimaginable energetic force. As your weight sinks downwards, be open to this force rushing upwards through your legs to meet it.

Be sensitive and you'll feel the meeting of the descending weight and the up-rushing telluric energy occurring somewhere just below your navel or thereabouts, engendering a swooshing-whooshing sensation akin to the power of two ocean currents meeting.

The Taoists call this region the sea of energy for this very reason and prescribe thinking, communicating and moving from it, using the swooshing-whooshing sensation therein as your physical driving force at all times, if you want to feel constantly supported, no matter what.

Discreetly let your upper body undulate, gyrate, sway and rock from the hips within your skin in a circular motion for a bit and feel the movement being instigated from just below your navel. Observe it happening from the center of your brain, breathing freely all the while, with your spine elongated and your weight sunk and you've entered the outer portals of hyper-reality.

Meanwhile, back in the hall of mirrors…

PURE theater

We're all acting here.

All of this – you, me and everyone else – it's nothing but theater making itself up as it goes along, according to prescribed patterns dictated at the start of time when this whole illusion began. This doesn't mean it isn't without its slings and arrows or that it doesn't hurt when you fall foul of them. The pain is what makes it convincing theater, just as is the pleasure.

In one act you're obliged to play the hero, the next act the anti-hero. One act you're the squeaky-clean one, the next you're all covered in dirt. One act you're winning, the next you're losing. And it swings round and round. This doesn't mean you're acting as someone else. On the contrary, in order to play the role with full effect, you have to be acting purely as you.

There is purity in the soul of every sentient being. That purity is the Tao.

You can access and touch it and by doing so repeatedly, be it. When you do, you are expressing the Tao in all your thoughts, words and deeds and the surface effect, the visible aspect of the role you're playing – visible both to yourself and others – will be pure: pure theater.

All reality is subjective, as far as each of us is concerned – the perception of which is all determined, as previously stated, by the stories we're telling ourselves about it. The only reality that comes anywhere close to being objective is when you're not in the way, when you're experiencing a moment of pure consciousness – but even then, as any quantum physicist will tell you, your very presence as an observer is transforming that which is being observed.

Everything is pure theater.

You're the co-creator. You're the co-director. You're the actor. You're part of the audience. And you're one of the people selling the ice creams. Above all, you're the Tao. And it's not as if you have any choice in it. The theater goes on whether you believe in it or not.

With approximately six and a half billion other people all vying for a set of rapidly dwindling resources along with you, the persistent nature of the theater is inevitable, at least while we still have this planet as our common home.

However, essentially, enjoying and therefore thriving on it all boils down to breathing in and out and being here in the moment, with all aspects of you organized, collected and marshalled into some kind of recognizable shape and unified force most of the time.

And being here requires making contact with the ground beneath your feet, as that's about the most physical phenomenon you can encounter and associate with.

You have to ground your pureness in physical reality, otherwise it remains a concept in your head – a mere intellectual conceit.

Assuming you have managed to make contact with the ground by sinking your weight and have simultaneously managed to keep your spine elongated, while breathing freely and gazing out at the world within and around you from the center of your brain, the next thing you'll be wanting by which to milk the high further, is a whisky-like sensation of warmth around your chest to act as an antidote to the fear of others messing up the play for you.

Am I resonating so far?

That's a rhetorical question, of course, and one I can only really answer myself at this point.

I believe I am.

And that's the best I can do right now.

As for the best you can do...

PURE heart

Your beating heart – your personal metronome, your rhythm meter – the driving core of your engine room and the font of your love and passion, that which gives your life its tone and value, ironically, is something words don't work for. The heart consciousness (for it is the seat of the mind, according to those old Taoists of yore) is beyond words. The consciousness of the heart is love. It's the aforementioned whisky-like feeling, a sensation of softness, warmth, harmony and safety arising whenever you relax your chest. Not in isolation, for that would be just a disconnected chest in a state of relaxation (and big deal, we've all seen disconnected chests in a state of relaxation and in themselves they do nothing to add to the fun) – but when you consciously connect your chest to the rest of you, keeping your gaze steady from the observation post in the center of your brain, your spine elongated and justified, the weight in your body sinking down below your navel and through your legs into the floor and the breath flowing freely in and out; and then relax the muscles all around the breastbone; it instantly alters your relationship with the external world for the better by injecting love into the mix. Love counters the fear you've been projecting unwittingly and, provided you keep it coming, no matter how the odds seem to be stacked against you out there in the big, bad world, events will swing round in your favour and keep doing so.

Love is the milieu in which miracles happen. Love is the soft side of the Tao and from softness derives true strength. Hardness makes you brittle and easy to snap. Softness makes you flexible and ultimately enduring and love will heal everything if you let it.

It's not an intellectual thing – not just some fanciful notion, to which you respond with an automatic smile and an 'Oh yes, love' feeling as if simply by saying so you've been a good person. It's something quite physical and has very little to do with being a good person.

For at the same time as you soften your chest, if you also gently raise your breastbone and visualize an opening in the center of the bone through which you're inhaling and exhaling directly, within a few breath cycles you'll notice an actual, active sensation of tingling warmth and wellbeing emerging from deep in your heart and radiating all about your person.

And while this in no way will prevent moments of disharmony and miscommunication between you and others – these are inevitable and necessary in terms of providing a viable contrast to harmony and effective communication – it will ensure all distortions in your relationship to the external world will resolve and heal over time. Moreover, by practicing awareness of the heart, as explained here, the incidence of miraculous resolutions between you and others will increase in frequency and intensity on an exponential basis – the more love you spread, the thicker and faster the miracles come.

PURE illusion

That's all this is – this book, you, me, everything you see around you, everything you think of as being around you; all of it. That doesn't mean it isn't here. It's here, or at least something is or we wouldn't be discussing it now, but it's not as it appears and is, generally speaking, the opposite of how it appears.

How does this help you? Information is power and the extent to which you're not entirely fooled by the illusion is the extent to which you're empowered. What's here is a coil of rope. What you're seeing is a snake. You think the snake is real and that its bite will kill you, but it's not a snake. All that's here is a coil of rope. The snake depends on the rope's existence for its own, as far as your perception is concerned, but the rope does not depend on the snake for its.

In other words, the atoms and molecules create form and forms come and go as the atoms and molecules continue their eternal dance, but the significance and value you give them and all phenomena associated with them depends entirely on you, so that ultimately even the notion that death is the worst thing that can happen to you, which is the case with most of us, no matter how enlightened we like to think we are, is actually subjective. The notion that you as an individual form have specific or particular value to the universe is ultimately merely subjective. So yes, the pain of injury or loss is real – it hurts. There's no denying that. And hurt is as real an experience as you can get. But the very idea that the you who experiences this hurt is anything more than a collection of habits that's become addicted to itself, and so thinks it's real, is deluded.

Of course, you'd defend your realness and argue with the preceding statement as any apparently sane person would; however, you know deep down you'd be wrong. That's the point of the charade. We all collude in reinforcing the notion that we are ultimately important, when any cemetery stands in directly contradictory proof.

Yes, you honor and respect the illusion of the snake – for being an illusion, not for being the rope itself, not ultimate reality. You honor and respect the fact that if when in snake-guise it bites you, it hurts, and can bring this dream to a sudden end; but you do so against a gestalt of knowing the whole show, including you, is nothing more than pure illusion.

This may or may not help you. There's nothing to resolve about it. It's a paradox. It's messy. Knowing that doesn't prevent the pain of being hurt but it helps you retain equilibrium knowing the theatre doesn't impinge on the purity of who you really are because that's universal, that's the Tao, hence limitless, hence invulnerable. The simple act of acknowledging this affords you a brief interlude in eternal time in which to know your pure self – maybe no more than a nano-second, but that's enough to gain a foothold.

It would be awfully slick if you could read a book, think about what's in it for a moment and be suddenly enlightened for ever more but it doesn't work like that. You have to meditate. You have to train. You have to make mistakes. You have to get confused. You have to find clarity. You have to doubt the methods. You have to prove them. You have to feel them gradually working their way through your system and transforming you from your deepest circuit boards outwards, and that takes time. Time and application. So I won't kid you. This purity we're after is a lifetime's process, but what's propounded in this book provides a viable start.

And so does recognizing that this book, you, me, everyone and everything you see (and think about) is an illusion. That doesn't mean it – they – isn't/aren't here at all. It is here but not as you're seeing or experiencing it. Argue with that if you enjoy arguing, otherwise bear with me and let's see if we can't make some sense of it as we go along. I doubt we will, because there really is no sense in any of it. Life is beyond any sense of sense we can appreciate with our rational minds, but I'm writing on till the end of the book anyway, so stay with me here unless you've got something better to do.

PURE trance

You are entranced. If you're reading this, you're entranced by the words, by the idea that this collection of pages comprises a book, that the book contains something you don't yet possess that you can download onto your mental hard drive, that downloading something you haven't got is good, that you and the importance of you are something as real as steel, that all of this, the world around you, the other people in your life, the ups and downs of fortune apparently at the hands of those around you and the idea that any of it matters, is all part of a trance. The traffic system, the financial system, the tax system, the banking system, the political system, the business system, the legal system, the international travel system, the air traffic control system – you're entranced by it all. You imagine this is reality but it's just a trance you're in.

What we're doing here is exchanging that trance, the trance of the everyday, for the trance of something deeper.

I don't quite know what it is. It's beyond words. I called it hyper-reality. I called it heaven. I called it the Tao but as I said, these are just words. I'm using words to get beyond words. I'm experimenting. And if you're still with me here, you're experimenting with me.

I'm always banging up against walls/rules doing that.

We all are.

There are no rules other than the ones we set ourselves, no walls other than those we build but every now and then, you bang up against one – some facet or other of the illusion that blocks your path – and you realize you've been momentarily outwitted by the illusion again.

But then you realize it's you who's creating the illusion in the first place.

Then you get dismayed because you doubt you'll ever find the keys to that layer of self that is creating the illusion so you can get to stop blocking your own path and create it differently.

That's why you're reading this book.

And why I'm writing it.

To hand you the keys.

But I don't really know if it's going to work.

How could I?

At the time of writing, I haven't written it yet.

So, in a way, you could dismiss any claims I made earlier.

I was just trying to entrance you.

And that's fair enough.

If I hadn't managed to entrance you we wouldn't have reached this stage where I'm forced to admit I haven't got a clue what I'm doing here or whether I have the ability to use words to get beyond words to the promised state of hyper-reality.

I have the ability to be there myself. I'm here now. I have to be to write like this.

And I will certainly present you the mechanics of how I do it, as I've been doing till now.

But whether I can make it come alive for you in a way that has its due impact, I don't yet know and nor do you.

That's the fun of it.

That's what makes it exciting.

My hunch is that I can, of course, or I wouldn't be bothering and nor would you.

How does it feel so far, meanwhile?

PURE cheek

So here I come along, convincingly telling you that nothing is as you think it is, not even you, and then I compound the confusion by confessing I don't know what I'm talking about. That's cheeky.

But so what.

It's true – assuming you go along with the original notion that what you experience of reality is a direct result of the story you're telling yourself about reality. And in any case, we've all become way too scared of offending each other these days by being a bit cheeky and that's silly – we've become soppy.

Meanwhile, I'm telling you you're hallucinating and that's cheeky.

But it grabs your attention and that's what it's all about. Wherever your attention goes, you can cause reality to shift.

So we started by gathering the mind in the central brain region. The attention went there and a shift occurred within you. Next, and not in any particular order, as they're all as important as each other, we spoke about the breathing, about lengthening the spine, sinking the weight, softening the chest and raising the breastbone – and as we did that, our attention went there together, so to speak, and a shift occurred in the way we each felt.

I'm assuming.

Read back if you dare and check out those points in detail again. I don't wish to big them up out of all proportion but these basic principles, which form the bedrock of this book and of the finer aspects of Taoist practice in general, comprise nothing less than the keys to hyper-reality, to enlightenment, to inner peace and to anything you wish to manifest in material reality. So don't just dismiss them as nothing special. The value you afford them will directly affect the value you get from them.

However, without relaxation, none of them is worth bothering with. Without relaxation you can't fully enter the hyper-reality sanctum. Tension constricts the flow of energy in your system and this snags the collective energy field for light years around, on account of which the guardians of hyper-reality keep the doors shut to you. Which is a lazy, fanciful way of saying you prevent yourself entering on account of being too distracted by your tension and, hence, you are too stiff to flow in through the crack (between the worlds).

And as relaxation is a much-misunderstood phenomenon, I'd like to attempt to clear it up for you.

PURE relaxation

Relax.

What do you do when I say that?

Think of tropical beaches and cocktails in the sun?

Think of watching the TV with your feet up?

Chill out.

How do you do that?

Ease off.

How's it done?

It's all in the muscles.

Take a moment to feel your muscles.

Touch some.

Squeeze your upper arm.

Feel the biceps.

Say, 'Hello, biceps'.

Don't expect the muscle to answer back, just imagine it.

Allow this childlike approach to make you aware of all your other muscles too. Feel your triceps, your forearm muscles, the muscles at the back of your neck, the muscles in your face, your throat, your chest, your shoulders, your upper back, your belly, your middle back, your pelvis, your lower back, your buttocks, your thighs, your calves, your shins and all the small muscles in your hands, feet and anywhere else I've forgotten to mention.

If you can't feel them, ask yourself why not.

They're your muscles.

The only reason you may think you can't feel them at will is because you've bought into a story you've told yourself that you can't feel them.

Stop all that for a moment and feel them now – all up and down and round your body from head to toe.

What are you doing with them all?

Check to see if you're gripping with them, where no gripping is actually required.

Negotiate with each muscle group in turn by explaining to each that the whole of you, including your muscles, will feel a lot better, healthier, springier, more positive, more effective, more alive and more comfortable, as soon as they stop gripping and let go.

Gradually induce your entire body to stop gripping and let go – and not just your muscles and sinews: relax your breathing, relax your blood flow, relax your organs, relax your bowels, relax your brain, relax your nervous system, relax your mind and finally relax your bones, at which point you can be said to have relaxed.

There's always further to go, mind, for as soon as you've achieved relaxation at one level, you'll instantly be aware of the next level of gripping that needs to stop and so on.

And it's good that it's so, for were it not for the tendency to grip and resist, you'd stop functioning altogether. So the tension serves a useful purpose. It's an aspect of the yin, the addictive. However, you don't have to concern yourself generally with upholding tension levels, as these will always be present on account of your innate fear of not surviving, so you're fairly safe in assuming that no matter how much you manage to relax, there'll always be another layer of tension to counterbalance it and prevent you dissolving.

It's a trick you're playing on yourself and it works.

I went up in a helicopter in Glasgow once. An old guy was flying it. He had the air of a man prone to a sudden heart attack. As we flew over breathtaking scenes of the Highlands, my visual rapture was heavily tempered by fear that the OG would die and I wouldn't have a clue how to fly the helicopter. I'd checked his moves a bit and had tried to glean the general idea but would not have fancied my chances of landing safely.

I noticed I was gripping on unconsciously to the edge of the seat. As soon as I noticed this I realized it was stupid, as no matter how hard I was gripping the seat, it would be of no avail should he die and we crash. So I tried to relax my grip, to let go

81

of the muscles and was amazed at how hard it was to do in spite of knowing how futile it was to grip on. I managed in the end by inching my way into it – a little bit of letting go, a little bit more gripping, a little bit more letting go and so on. Eventually I relaxed all the way but by then the ride was over and we were landing.

That's kind of how it is with you in your life. So I empathize with how hard it is to achieve this simple feat of desisting from gripping needlessly with the muscles.

Nonetheless, you have to start somewhere and now's as good a point as any, especially if you don't want to leave it all the way till the end of the ride.

Conversely, that idea of having only finally relaxed once you're landing is also a good metaphor for the dynamic whereby the sooner you relax about whatever or whomever it is you're perceiving as threatening your survival in some way, the sooner it or they stop being an actual threat, if indeed they ever really were one.

We imagine lots of things, some of which may even be accurate at the time, but forms, people and atmospheres change as quickly as the wind, relatively speaking, so there's no need to credit external phenomena with too much power over you. Indeed, following the principles in this book, you stand every chance of gaining access to hyper-reality in which you take command of externals from within rather than vice versa.

I'm not selling it to you too heavily, as I know full well that even with the best methods in the universe, which I believe these are among, you still find yourself becoming confused and filled with doubt at times.

Of course you do.

You're creating scenarios to provide you with the stimulus for doing just that – confusing yourself and hence giving way to doubt.

And why?

Because evidently you enjoy it.

PURE confusion

You are creating all the adversity in your life – no one and nothing else is – and you can stop blaming yourself for it now. It's not a crime. It can be fun having obstacles to overcome. Why make it easy if you can make it difficult? I can see why you enjoy that. I do it myself from time to time. So you create blocks to overcome and to give the storyline more shape and substance. However, you confuse yourself by subscribing to the belief that just because you're confusing everyone else by appearing to be a victim and thus influencing them to play the same game, and thus perpetrating a spread of victim-minded confusion far and wide, you also deserve to be confused by yourself into believing you're a victim too.

And, if you find that confusing or feel that I'm in some way abusing your mind, I'll just keep it simple and say that you'll find, from this very day, nothing will ever be the same again, providing you take this opportunity to acknowledge it's you who are creating the blockages to your perfect happiness; nothing and nobody else. All the outside is doing is colluding with you in a pretense, a charade, a bit of theatre. Which is fine, but it's time to go deeper now.

Clarity consists entirely in you knowing that you're in command of the theater of your life.

Be confused no longer.

As soon as you acknowledge yourself as story-creator and give thanks to all external players for playing their part, knowing that in each is the same divine spark that ignites your own soul, the apparent external adversity will be dispelled in real time – it will cease to have any effect on your progress.

You are then free to create it differently from here.

But you can't even begin to do that when you're confused about who or what it is doing it.

Acknowledge the confusion.

Acknowledge yourself for creating it.

Acknowledge that you're enjoying it – this includes enjoying not enjoying it.

Own it fully.

Don't blame yourself.

You've done nothing wrong in creating this confusion. It was fine doing that, but now it's time for clarity. You want clarity.

So you don't even bother fighting the idea that much.

Instead, take a moment or more now to consider all the scenarios in your life that you perceive as obstacles to your progress in manifesting your perfect happiness, along with all the external conditions required to facilitate that happiness in real time.

Consider all the people actually or potentially involved.

Realize that each is merely obeying signals you're sending out, unconsciously, to collude with the dramatic stance you've been adopting till now. Realize each is merely playing his, her or its part in the theater you've set up of being a victim. Realize you've been enjoying it. Mentally thank them sincerely for playing their parts so willingly and adroitly, then move on by asking yourself how you'd like the action to go from here.

PURE choice

So you've settled your consciousness in the center of your brain, given your spine a bit of length, softened your muscles, got your breathing to flow more freely, allowed your weight to sink below your navel, opened your heart to let your love flow, have allowed in notions of the Tao and how it expresses itself theatrically in your life, have started taking responsibility for having manifested things the way they are and have now reached the point of being able to choose where you want the story to go from here, in terms of the outcome and the tone of the experience along the way.

In fact, attending to all of the above in the first place constitutes your primary choice. Once you've made the choice to settle fully into yourself and take command, all the rest will follow on naturally anyway.

However, to help it along and nudge it in what looks like an appealing direction (for you never know till you try it), it will serve you to choose the outcome you wish for from the next foreseeable phase and the tone in which you wish to experience it as you go along.

For instance, for you the next phase might be the upcoming three-month period, the outcome of which you'd like to be, say, you having overcome whatever obstacles seem to be in your way just now, having achieved something great that will have ameliorated conditions for you in all respects, including having manifested greater abundance and finding yourself immensely joyful of heart for having beautiful people close to you with all manner of blessings on your head. And you might wish to experience everything that occurs between now and then to facilitate that in a relaxed, centered, cheerful, confident, collected, loving way, thus lending a relaxed, centered, cheerful, confident, collected, loving tone to the experience.

So, from your control tower in your center brain and with all your body aligned, relaxed and optimally arranged and poised beneath, you see all these as if they are projected onto a screen before you. See yourself in the scene, being that person. Then, with the fullness of yourself, declare mentally or aloud as appropriate, 'I choose this.' At this point, note that that person in the scene is you and you are that person and allow yourself to feel the sensation of being that person, which shouldn't be too hard as you are that person.

You'll notice your attention flickering on and off it. And that's fine and natural.

Providing during the moments of flickering on it, you're seeing it clearly enough, this will instigate an irreversible process leading to you being that person within the allotted timeframe, or thereabouts.

Pretty much the only thing that could throw a spanner in the works at this point is your belief that you don't deserve it, that you're not worthy. But even that cannot fully get in the way of you now attracting what you want to you.

Belief in your own unworthiness is merely another theatrical device you use to confuse yourself with, fueled by the illusion of victim-hood. It's fine to indulge it as long as you find it helps you in some way. It can even be quite fetching to feign unworthiness sometimes. But it's bullshit.

PURE Interference

Running interference on yourself, thereby causing external reality to copy you and run interference on you in real time, is an addictive pattern, and inasmuch as any addiction has its enjoyable moments, it is occasionally an engrossing thing to do to yourself. Like self-harming with a razor blade, it has its romantic charm in a deeply distorted, twisted way. However, were you to stop, you'd probably find that more enjoyable still. Interference, or static, arises from that aspect of you that has bought into the story that you're unworthy of achieving what you want. This gives rise to self-doubt at every turn, which is also enjoyable in a self-harming way but uses up a lot of energy and leaves you drained of the power you actually need to get on with the actual everyday work required to make your life be as you want it to be. As well as which, by instigating and perpetuating a fearful thought-form, it eventually draws to you the very thing you fear most, so is ultimately self-defeating.

And though your rational adult mind knows this and is almost insulted by it being stated, so obvious is it, the unconscious part of you where you've been hiding this belief in self-defeat is strangely unwilling to give up the game. Indeed, it has even ascribed itself an illusory personality based on performing this task on a regular basis, so it is bound to uphold the status quo for its survival – until you tell it to stop.

This split-off part of you must now be induced back into the fold on a fully cooperative basis, so that you can move forward in the story less encumbered.

You need to be light now.

You need to know that with every step you take from now on, you're growing lighter and lighter, freer and freer.

You can no longer afford to be weighed down with doubt, you can no longer afford your progress be stayed by interference you're running on your own self.

Initially, even though in your rational mind you realize it's you who's running the interference, it feels impossible that you'd be able to stop it – it's simply too big and difficult to tackle. It's foolhardy to even dare think about it.

However, it is only a habit and no matter how much you kid yourself you like doing it, it really isn't that enjoyable. There isn't even a high – just a long, drawn-out, niggling low.

Imagine reaching your last breath and wondering why you wasted all that precious, beautiful time here on the planet believing you were obliged to make yourself stressed over nothing, when you could have simply been enjoying it.

What makes you feel obliged to do that to yourself?

PURE Nonsense

You believe you're not good enough. You believe you have something to be ashamed of. You believe you're inferior. You believe you're a fraud. You believe you're unworthy. You believe you're incapable. Which is all pure nonsense.

You're neither good enough nor bad enough. You have nothing to be ashamed of and everything to be ashamed of. You're as behind as you are in front. You're as real as you're fake. You're as deserving as you're undeserving and you're as capable as you're incapable. These are all just opinions, based on spurious, subjective, relative criteria and they ultimately mean nothing.

Assume that if you managed to assume the form you're in, along with all your ineffable talents and skills, in a universe where the odds of doing so and sustaining it successfully this long are too great to fit in this book, you are good enough; you have enough to feel proud about, you are authentic enough, you are deserving enough and you are capable enough to achieve anything less – less here referring to all the remaining details comprising the various aspects of your existence you'd like to change or improve.

If you're good enough to make it into human form and be evolved enough along the path to be sitting, standing, lying or crouching here reading this, you're generally enough and can be fairly confident in your chances of achieving whatever it is you want, no matter how big or complex.

One thing you can be sure of is you're good enough, respectable enough, on-the-level enough, real enough, deserving enough and capable enough to dismantle this insane belief that you're none of these things and to do so this very instant.

How?

Stop thinking about all this for a minute now. Thinking about all this too much only gives you a headache and achieves nothing. This wisdom isn't to do with thinking. It's to do with being purely you.

Return to the basic set-up.

Draw your mind back into the center of your brain. Lengthen your spine. Breathe slowly and low down – allowing your belly to swell on inhalation and exhale on exhalation. Sink all your weight below your navel. Relax all your muscles and sinews – stop gripping onto nothing. Soften your chest to allow your love to stream freely, smile with your eyes and just be here until you read the next word...........

that's better.

Realize that in this state you are no longer bound by the limited conception you had of yourself. You are no longer laboring under the illusion that your being was enclosed in your skin. Your physical form is now merely the access point through which to locate your center but your center, and all the rest of you, is universal in scale and scope. The physical is now just the metaphor you've become habituated to latching onto for the sake of description. And that's lazy.

In the same way that you find it hard to experience life from within the tip of the big toe on your left foot, unless you stub it, so you find it hard to experience life from within any other point in this vast, limitless universe. But you are the farthest star as much as you are the inside of the tip of your left big toe.

I'm selling you the story that you're universal and unbounded here and that the only reason you argue with that is because you've bought into a different story that says you stop at your skin.

Are you buying it?

You don't have to answer that.

It doesn't matter.

However, instead of entering a debate about whether it matters or not, or whether indeed it's valid in the first place, suspend rational judgment and indulge a brief mental flight of fancy to the farthest reaches of your imagination – far, far beyond the most distant galaxy, a billion, zillion light years hence.

Rather than having got here by zooming like a human missile through space, you've arrived here simply by expanding your sense of self – like blowing up an airbed bigger and bigger – until you burst beyond the confines of your skin and rapidly grow larger than your town, region, country, continent, hemisphere, planet, solar system, galaxy, universe and are now finally so large you're containing everything that is – and are rapidly expanding to include even more still.

Consider yourself the ultimate entity now.

Could there possibly be anything about you as the ultimate entity (the Tao) that is unworthy or deficient in any way, and if so, who is there to judge? You contain it all and everyone in it, so who's to judge you?

You are a version of the Tao. The Tao is you. You are the Tao. The Tao does not criticize itself. You criticizing yourself and then living your life according to that critique is like the Tao criticizing itself. You are encouraging the Tao to do that and that causes it discomfort by creating too limiting and inane a state. So stop now – it's rude. Let the Tao be as big as it wants – universal – and remember you are the Tao and the Tao is you.

Let yourself be as big as you want.

Let yourself be as powerful as you want.

Let yourself be as capable as you want.

Let yourself be as deserving as you want.

Let yourself be as real as you want.

Let yourself be as successful as you want.

Let yourself be as rich as you want.

Let yourself be as popular as you want. Let yourself be as loveable as you want. And above all, let yourself be.

That's it.

Let yourself be.

You are the Tao.

The Tao lets itself be.

If it didn't, none of this would be here – it wouldn't be happening.

The Tao lets itself be this.

Let yourself be this.

Say, 'I am this.'

Stop getting in the way with nonsensical beliefs about not being enough now.

You're enough.

OK, that's enough of that now.

PURE Elegance

Do you know what you want?

When you relax and come out of the noise in your forebrain and look at your life from the center of your brain, do you see what it is you want?

When you cast your awareness into your belly and chest, can you feel what you want?

Can you feel anything there?

What are you feeling?

Excitement?

Fear? Inertia? Agitation? Peace?

Love? Contentment? Perturbation? Stillness?

Warmth? Cold? Weakness? Strength?

A combination?

Nothing?

What pictures arise in your forebrain as you feel what you're feeling there?

Keep breathing.

What pictures are you seeing?

Just focus on the happy ones for now – leave the others for another time.

What are the happy pictures you're seeing?

Where do you see yourself?

How are you looking? What are you wearing? What are you doing?

Whatever it is, that's one of the things you want.

Each time you do it you'll see something else you want.

That's how you find out what you want.

The rest of it is mostly imaginary.

Things you think you want, or think you should still want because you started wanting them a long time ago, or because others have wanted them for you for a long time, or because you've never had any better ideas than those you've seen others have and have been clinging on to some hodgepodge mishmash of a visualization comprised of them by default – all of that can be discarded now.

It's true.

You don't have to hold onto whatever it is you've been wanting all this time unless you still want to.

You can create anything you want now.

But only if it's authentic.

Only if the desire to create it arises from the depths, as opposed to being superimposed from the surface realm of externally driven stimuli – only if it's original, only if it's authentic, only if it's pure.

Close the window on the chatter in the front of your brain, step back a bit, into the center of your brain. Below, let your body go. Feel what you're feeling. Do all the moves you've picked up so far in the book – read it again, if you need to refresh your mind; I'll still be here. Attend to the spine, the body, the breathing and all, and drop into the hyper-real zone with me here and let the pictures come – let them arise out of the void visible between and behind your eyes when you lower your lids and feel what you're feeling in the belly and chest.

Ignore any pictures that make you feel awkward, sad, miserable, scared or at odds and keep focusing from way back in the center of your brain into the void behind your eyes until your gaze picks out the happy picture or pictures arising there. At this point, desist from allowing your rational mind to play devil's advocate. There is no legal or any other sort of obligation on your part to engage in playing devil's advocate with yourself and especially not now, when you're involving yourself in creating your life from scratch here.

This is important business and you need all the positive support from yourself you can muster. Override the internal criticism at this point, therefore, and allow all the arising pictures that make you happy to make you happy, without getting in the way and spoiling the moment.

Sometimes the pictures are direct messages, sometimes metaphors.

You may see yourself in a palace you own on some hill overlooking some city somewhere in the world, the twinkling lights below, feeling as fine as fine can be, having achieved whichever remarkable feat it is you're wanting to achieve just now, feeling literally on top of the world. That could mean you actually want that to occur in real time, or that you want to feel fine as fine and to know yourself as the king or queen of your world as it is now, even if you actually live in the dip of a valley in a two-up, two-down.

Either way, it doesn't matter and you'll get it. It doesn't matter because the feeling is the experience and the rest are details you can then go on to refine. There might be elements of the palace you want to incorporate in the valley house or the palace might be symbolic of a palace of a different kind, somewhere different from where you imagined it – the variables are endless.

As you allow yourself to feel yourself being that person, feeling that way, you create a magnetic field of that quality of feeling which attracts to you phenomena of a similar tone, which by and by come into a state of manifestation, always with a twist, of course, as that's the nature of reality on account of the play of yin and yang driving it all along – there's a shaft of shade for every streak of light and a shaft of light for every streak of shade.

And that's fine too.

Witness the unfolding of your manifestation in real time as an example of pure elegance.

Elegance as an expression of perfection implies imperfection, without which it would have nothing to be contrasted with.

Were you ever to achieve the perfect manifestation, you'd have reached the stage where yin and yang were no longer operating in your life and you would either be an immortal in human form or a bullshitter. It's why Chuang Tsu, the second quasi-official forefather of the Taoist quasi-tradition, sometimes referred to the Tao, the ineffable presence behind all this, as the Great Swindler – there's always another side to every story.

Hence none of it matters.

And it all matters.

At least you think you do. But all opinions are relative. Rest your mind now.

Transcend the realm of preferences. Return awareness to your breathing. Slow it down.

Align yourself and relax as prescribed and we'll go deeper into refining the manifesting process.

PURE Depth

Depth is perceptual and relative. How deep is deep? However deep you go you can always go a lot deeper.

What is deep anyway?

Deep is essentially nothing.

Go deep enough into the ground and you come out on the other side of the planet again – you arrive back at the surface. The whole process – every process – is circular.

You think it's highly superficial of you to like someone just because they have a nice face. But if you look behind the surface to the associations your unconscious has made between that face and pleasant infantile memories or thought impressions you may have, and then look behind that to the vulnerability of you as an infant and all the implications of having become one in the first place – the love or otherwise between your mother and father and where they were coming from in terms of associations and just about everything else involved – you will realize there's nothing shallow about liking someone because of their face at all. And what's not deep about a face? For though it's on the front surface of the skull and therefore easy to brush off as a superficial layer or covering – there to stop your nose falling off or your eyes falling out – if you had to create an authentic living face from scratch you'd be defeated before you began, so profound is the process that actually does create one. Go deep enough with all of yourself, into pure depth, and the depth becomes shallow – this is an example of how pure cancels out the illusion.

So there's nothing intrinsically deep about deep and if you follow deep to its extreme you come back to the surface anyway. However, in this world of illusions where we create something out of nothing and call it the world, we thrive on relativity. We thrive on the illusion that deep is deep and can positively use it to help anchor our intention to be or do something, in a psychic zone that seems to have more depth than the everyday trance state – hyper-reality – and by doing so, we are able to inform the intention with the power to manifest it as some form of beneficial change of circumstances and conditions in real time.

In other words, anchor an intention to the core of your being and you invest it with the power to bear actual fruit in the world for you.

The core of your being is not tangible, as you know. If someone were to cut into you, all the way to the core of your physical body, your spine, they would still not find you there. However, the spine serves as a physical metaphor for the core of your being and by anchoring your intention to it by the following internal maneuver you'll be able to purify and refine it to a strong enough essence to manifest pretty much anything your heart desires.

You must bear in mind, when doing this, that manifesting whatever your heart desires brings with it a whole universe you might not have been counting on having to deal with – a plethora of new responsibilities you didn't have before. This is unlikely to stop you going for it, though, and there's no reason you should fight the evolutionary thrust of existence and resist it.

Evolution consists of making something out of nothing. At first there was nothing. Nothing by virtue of its very existence implied its opposite, something – otherwise how could it be at all? The one became two and the universe was born and continues being born by an exponential proliferation of series of steps of making something out of nothing and refining that something till it creates the illusion of a world without end, hence why it's hard putting the brakes on this illusion simply because we realize we haven't got the resources to sustain it. It hurts when illusions of permanence get shattered. The unrest and violence we now see in the world result from the pain of the illusion being shattered before we've had time to create a better one.

That's why this information is coming through for us now. The universal mind knows it's time for us to create a new illusion and is making more knowledge available to us to help us do that – even though it is us and we are it – while we're in the illusion we're playing hide-and-seek with it and it with us.

Go with all that if you will. Don't, if not. It doesn't matter. It's not necessarily true. It's simply a stance.

However, the maneuver in question will take you beyond abstraction to the nub of the manifesting process. It comprises you tuning in to your spine and visualizing an orbital loop beginning between your legs, rising up the rear of your spinal column over the top of your brain and then descending down the frontal aspect of your spine and down between your legs to complete the circuit.

When nothing became something and started proliferating in ones and zeros till we had the world we see around us now, it was following the basic dance of yin and yang – negative (nothing) and positive (something). These two opposite and complementary forces also run through your body. By tapping into their flow you tap into the essential pre-atomic evolutionary thrust of existence itself and that's what gives your magic its power.

The ascending aspect of the loop is the main channel for the yang force. The descending aspect is the main channel for the yin.

The yin force is all about things becoming nothing – all about reduction or purification. The yang force is all about nothing becoming something – all about increase or refining what is.

Go on to visualize a fine, yet limitlessly powerful, stream of pure white light rising slowly up the rear aspect, going over the top of the brain and dropping equally slowly through the frontal aspect.

Gradually allow your breathing rhythm to slow down and fall into the same tempo as the rise and fall of the light. Inhale as the light ascends, exhale as it descends.

As the light travels upwards it refines the story you're telling yourself about reality – it refines your reality, in other words. As the light descends, it purifies the story and your resulting reality.

Refining means to make stronger by increasing the inbound flow of energy, force, people and resources. Purifying means paring away all extraneous elements and cleansing yourself of all aspects that have been causing hindrance to the refining process. They're a hair's-breadth apart but the distinction is worth making.

As the light travels round the loop in time with your breath, think about what you're intending. For example, you may be intending the outcome of today to be one of pure joy and feeling purely at one with yourself and all the world, and for that to result in a run of beautiful surprises coming your way over the next couple of days or so. Once identified, take that intention, insert it in the flow of light and let it circulate approximately nine times, feeling it becoming progressively more refined and purified with each successive orbit.

Watch it all from the center of your brain. Keep breathing. Keep your spine elongated. Sink your weight. Relax all your muscles and sinews. Raise your breastbone and soften your chest.

You can apply this no matter the complexity or intricacy of the outcome you intend, or of the time frame involved.

However, always expect the unexpected.

One of your mind's favorite addictions is imagining it has a handle on guessing how the future's going to be. It likes to play out reality in your imagination before it's happened. It bases its models on what's gone before. Because the future is the result of the ongoing exponential proliferation of something being made out of nothing, it's impossible for your past experience to include all the necessary information upon which to base a model equipped to deal with the exponentially expanded reality the future will comprise. Rehearsing from models like this limits your range and scope of conceptualizing and manifesting what you want, as you'll just be running on old patterns so you won't manifest anything new – it all might look different but will result in the same old story of discontent.

Instead, use that aspect of mind to concentrate on sitting in anticipation of surprises.

Shout the sound HAH! suddenly.

See, you didn't know that was coming, and nor did anyone around you.

Let life surprise you now.

Don't be afraid or superstitious. It won't go bad on you unless you want it to.

Get clear with yourself about the outcome you desire now – keep it as broad as possible. For example, you may desire an outcome that sees you suddenly able to feel more relaxed than you've ever felt before about absolutely everything and that by attaining that blissful state you induce the gods and spirits to shower you with unexpected blessings of all sorts. You don't know what they'll be. You don't need to know what they'll be. You just know they'll be.

Then you settle back, do what you have to do in earth-plane reality – perhaps carry on reading this book for a while – and allow life to surprise you with the way things turn out.

You can specify the broad heading these surprises will fall under too. For example, you can specify surprises in connection with material abundance, career opportunities, relationship healings, physical healings, meeting new people to enrich your life, quantum leaps in development of skills or talents, or in fact anything you like. But don't specify the precise result – don't limit what can turn out by confining your own imagination. Allow the Tao to surprise you.

Or don't.

You can specify if you want; however, it will require a lot more energy to support the process and you will often find it doesn't match up to your expectations when you get it anyway.

The way of the game I'm presenting you – the game of wu wei – is the way of allowing yourself to be surprised. The results are invariably far huger that way.

When people talk about Taoism being about acquiescence, this is what they mean. Set your intention, anchor it to your core, and then let go and allow the Tao to surprise you.

This means you have to be innocent.

PURE Innocence

You are innocent. I'm innocent. Everyone is innocent. It doesn't matter what you've done. It doesn't matter what anyone has done.

What you are, what we all are, is innocence – pure innocence.

However, we obscure it from ourselves and each other by adding layers of disguises to give the appearance of being guilty of something. We then act out to justify that and so generate a living illusion of guilt. This is merely a device to separate ourselves from the Tao. This is what is meant by the Fall – the original sin – to indulge the arrogance of assuming a stance of being separate from and therefore even more powerful than the Tao. More powerful, because if the Tao is the universe and you are something apart from that, you must be even more powerful. So rather than thinking yourself humble to consider yourself a lowly creature in the face of the almighty Tao, consider yourself arrogant for it and instead acknowledge you are the Tao in human form. The Tao is guilty of nothing. The Tao is innocent and therefore so are you.

This doesn't mean you don't make mistakes. Everyone does. That's how we learn.

However, by focusing on guilt for the mistakes you've made, thus strengthening that as a thought-form, you're giving your mind the command to re-enact that pattern perpetually in one form or another. But by tuning into your innocence you make that the dominant thought-form and are hence naturally less and less inclined to act out guilt-inducing patterns in future.

There's no other way round it. Tune into your innocence now, thereby cleansing yourself of the shackles of outworn patterns.

PURE dedication

Without dedication, none of this means anything – not just the book but the whole story of your life – without dedication, none of it means anything. Things only mean something when you dedicate yourself.

What you dedicate yourself to is secondary. The primary factor is dedication to your life. It's a state of being. From there, you can apply your dedication to the aspects of life that draw your fascination and beg your engagement and commitment to remaining engaged for the duration, come what may, through all the rises and falls of keenness, through all the variations in ease and difficulty levels connected to your continuing engagement in those aspects.

What are you dedicated to? What are you dedicating yourself to?

What you dedicate yourself to expands and grows and bears fruit and causes changes in your circumstances. What you dedicate yourself to causes your life story to unfold. What you dedicate yourself to rewards you with abundance.

Some people are dedicated to feeling pain and distress. Some people are dedicated to giving pain and distress. For their dedication they will be rewarded by an abundance of pain and distress.

Some people are dedicated to feeling energy and joy. Some people are dedicated to giving energy and joy. They will be rewarded with an abundance of energy and joy.

Most people are dedicated to a combination, until they realize there's a choice involved and always was. At that point, they tend to remind themselves to dedicate themselves to feeling and giving energy and joy through every activity and avenue open to them and are then rewarded with an abundance of energy and joy.

This they then apply to the creative and material endeavors that draw their fascination and are rewarded with creative and material success.

But at the base of it all lies the requirement to dedicate yourself to your life, the nub of which is accessible deep in the core of your being through the meditation process.

Dedicate yourself to the meditation process and all other areas of dedication will bear fruit.

Meditate and you'll grow rich (in all ways), in other words.

Pure dedication is but a hair's-breadth distance from pure belief, and the distinction is worth making.

In a state of pure belief, you know you are manifesting what you want. In a state of pure dedication, you are fully harnessed to the process and are thus able to fulfil your obligations in connection with whatever you dedicate yourself to, with a cheerful heart, as an act of communion, rather than with resistance as an act of sufferance.

Dedication provides the link between you and others, through which your gift is able to be received and, therefore, by which you make your contribution to the world via your creative and material endeavors.

Dedication is a property of the heart. You feel it from there – you commit from there. Only then does it fully link you to the collective and to the Tao informing it, whence comes your reward of abundance of whatever it is you're dedicating yourself to.

Consciously dedicating the fruits of the meditation process, the fruits of being dedicated to your life, to others; actively dedicating the good feeling in your heart to those in need, exponentially amplifies the effects of practice, there and then in the moment. So, whenever you're practicing what's in this book, end the session by dedicating the feeling in your heart to those in need – this can extend to include all sentient beings, as there are very few of us not in need of some extra good feeling to help things along as we work, rest and play.

And while we're on endings, we must also address beginnings, as one follows the other as surely as yin follows yang, or night follows day. On starting a session of practicing any aspect of what's in this book, clarify what you're dedicated to – clarify what you wish to make manifest in your life, in other words. This act of book-ending the session with a motivation check and dedication makes it sacred – it makes it connect to the source of all being and power, whence springs the vital juice to make reality manifest into its new shape for you.

PURE success

Pure success is when you are not at odds with yourself, not fighting with yourself, not punishing yourself, not doing yourself down. It is when you are at peace with yourself, at peace with the force of life informing you: a unified entity, simultaneously at peace with the external world, or your perception of it, regardless of external conditions. Success, then, in its pure form, is about what's going on within you. It's another way of describing being purely you.

When you're experiencing pure success in this way, the external world reflects it back at you by showering you with the gifts your mind associates with success: career advancement, wealth accumulation, respect, renown and whatever other success symbols you've lodged in your unconscious.

When you are living in a state of pure success, in other words, you spontaneously manifest whatever you associate with success in the external world.

However, when this occurs, providing you choose to remain in the state of pure success and don't choose the option of allowing yourself to be suckered in and fooled by external appearances, the effects will merely be cause for an inner confirmatory smile of thanks, rather than becoming your reason for living.

The reward is in the internal state, rather than in the external symbols, and the surest way of ensuring your external success keeps growing is to train your focus to remain on the inner state of purity.

Of course, you'll flip in and out of it and the outside will reflect that by flickering lighter and darker, metaphorically speaking. The important thing is making sure you keep flipping in.

Meantime, success is all relative and no matter how pure or impure your state, or whether you're flipped in or flipped out, the propensity of external conditions to reflect your internal state means you will invariably be successful in manifesting the external reality you want.

The proof is all around you. What you perceive as your reality is the reality you've manifested so far. You have been successful at that. The fact there may be elements that displease you does not detract from this success.

However, during moments of experiencing the state of pure success, wherein you enter hyper-reality (as you do whenever you are in a pure state of any kind), you can direct the way the external reflects back at you.

But before you can expect your forays into hyper-reality to yield you the results you wish for, you have to begin by acknowledging your success so far, including your success at manifesting elements that displease you. Until you do that, you're stuck in a failure-oriented holding pattern.

You will succeed at manifesting whatever you want. Success is guaranteed.

Success is not an elusive substance that only comes to people with special powers or attributes.

Success is an intrinsic, pre-atomic aspect of the Tao and is available to everyone at all times, no matter what.

Success is a way of describing the mechanism whereby an intention becomes fact in real time.

Success and dedication are no more than a hair's-breadth apart, but the distinction is worth making. Whatever you dedicate yourself to, you'll successfully manifest in real time.

Dedication represents your commitment to manifesting it.

Success describes the part of the process whereby dedication transforms reality into something new.

Success does not discriminate between healthy and unhealthy intentions – it doesn't care whether you're dedicated to construction or destruction. It will oblige you either way.

Success is another way of describing the evolutionary force, which will find outlet through everyone, no matter what they're dedicated to.

Whereas dedication is a property of the heart, success in its pre-atomic form is a property of the solar plexus.

The more relaxed your solar plexus, therefore, the more freely your energy can flow there, the more instantly you manifest what you want.

But however fast or slow, everyone is eventually successful at manifesting what they want.

Whatever you intend, you will successfully manifest.

Knowing this, now is a perfect opportunity to reflect on what you're intending to manifest in the next phase.

At first, allow yourself to relax, especially in the solar plexus region, and drop into the internal zone as prescribed.

Note whatever your mind is afraid of. These fears generally fall under five main categories. Categorizing them is a viable method for beginning to deconstruct, and hence neutralize, them. First, there's the fear of not making a living. Second, there's the fear of having a bad reputation. Third, there's the fear of death and dying of anything other than old age. Fourth, there's the fear of hell, or as the Buddhists, who first made these categories, put it, the fear of being reborn into an evil life. And finally comes the fear of experiencing pain or unpleasant conditions of any kind during this lifetime.

When you identify a fear in any of the above categories, which you surely will, be aware that these represent unconscious desires until they are dragged out into the light of day and transformed into their opposite by conscious intention.

So, for instance, say you're afraid you'll lose your source of income for one reason or another, see the picture and transform it into one where you're unfailingly earning an ample living doing what you most enjoy. You don't even have to know how. You can leave that to the magical mechanics of the manifesting process – the wu wei of it. All you have to know is that money or wherewithal of any kind is merely a symbolic form of energy and that providing you're contributing your energy to the greater good, that energy will swing back round your way, multiplied in the form you need it most, and if that's money, you'll have money. Other than that, just let yourself see the picture of you feeling safe and secure earning an ample living doing what you most enjoy. Feel yourself being that person. Inhabit the body of that person. Believe it to be so in hyper-reality, trusting that what is real there will become real in everyday reality in due course. This will ensure a healthy flow of money in your direction at all times. Knowing that, you can now afford to relax. The more you relax, the more chi you have flowing through your channels. The more chi you have flowing in your channels, the more power your intention has. The more power your intention has, the faster and more significantly you'll manifest the reality you want, including having an ample living.

Or if you're afraid, for whatever reason, that you'll gain a bad reputation among your peers and those you perceive to count in your world, however few or many they are, see yourself respected and acknowledged for being the beautiful, unique expression of the Tao that you are. That's all you have to know: you are a beautiful, unique expression of the Tao in human form and the extent to which you identify with that is the extent the opinions of others will have an impact on you, in inverse proportion. Otherwise, see yourself respected for being purely you and once you can see what that looks like, feel it too. Feel what it's like inhabiting the body of that person who's respected for being purely them. Hold the sensation steady for a moment so it fixes itself in hyper-reality and know that once it is fixed there, it will also manifest in the everyday in the course of time. Or, if you're afraid of dying before your time, see yourself living to a ripe old age and finally releasing your mortal coil because you've truly had enough by then and are fully ready to move on to the next stage of soul-evolution. At the same time, see yourself passing gracefully and smoothly no matter when you die. All you have to know is that death is perfectly safe, that what you are is pure consciousness, energy and love in form, and that consciousness, energy and love are infinite – they've

122

always been present and always will be, forever and ever – they change form but are never depleted, so you, the essence of you, never dies. Otherwise, see yourself as that person fully ready to let go at any time in full trust that the ride is perfectly safe and see yourself like that at an old age. Once you can see the picture, allow yourself to feel it too. Feel what it's like to inhabit the body of that person crossing over in a state of absolute serenity and grace. Let the picture lodge in hyper-reality and know it will manifest like that in real time – hopefully a long, long way off in real time.

Or if you're afraid of being cast into eternal torment or coming back as, say, a prawn scuttling along the sea bed in a state of depression, see yourself entering the realm of the Golden Immortals as a radiant being of pure light with a universe-size smile on your celestial face, far beyond the mortal cares of this mundane reality. All you have to know is that's who you really are and always have been all the while anyway, so on dropping your body and the disguises that come with it, all the confusion will lift and you'll be who you always were anyway, but were too distracted to notice. Otherwise, see yourself as that Golden Immortal and when you can see it clearly, feel it too. Feel what it's like being unbounded and beyond the constraints of time or space. Allow that image to lodge in hyper-reality and know it will manifest. If, however, you reckon you won't be able to hack

123

it being in the undifferentiated state for eternity and will require distraction, see yourself being reborn into the life of someone extremely privileged in every respect on a planet somewhere that isn't threatened by overpopulation, where the disease of greed and envy hasn't yet taken hold. All you have to know is that all of it is a thundering great illusion, and from the state of hyper-reality you can bend that illusion any way you choose, providing your intention is steady enough. Otherwise, see the picture or succession of pictures and feel what it's like being that soul incarnating into a fabulous existence and thinking, 'Well done, me.' And that's what you'll manifest.

How do I know?

I don't.

And it doesn't matter. What matters is transforming fear into delight, without which you'll manifest what you fear, rather than what delights you.

Or if you have fear of experiencing pain, see yourself in a state of perpetual comfort and ease. All you have to know is that pain is just an opinion. Otherwise, see yourself feeling perpetual comfort in your skin and when you can see it, allow yourself to feel what it's like being in the body of that person in a state of perpetual comfort. Allow the image to lodge in hyper-reality and know it will come to pass in real time.

Then turn your attention to creating something new.

Start with the broad concept. For instance, you may be intending to manifest a reality in which you find yourself being authentic all the time – feeling and being free to express yourself as you will, surrounded with abundance, supported by great wealth, enjoying authentic loving relations with everyone close to you, basking in an atmosphere of harmony, without material cares or pressure in a state of glowing health. (This is merely an example; I'm not telling you what to want – only you know what that is.)

See yourself in the midst of whatever scene that conjures up in your mind. Watch yourself for a while enjoying it. Check out your clothes (assuming you're wearing some in the scene), examine the way your face looks, paying attention to the expression and zooming into the smile lines at the corners of your eyes. As you do this, allow yourself to feel what it's like being in your body (in the scene), allow yourself to feel what's going on in the chest and belly of that person. Allow yourself to smell the smells. Spend some time. Don't rush yourself. Listen to the sounds around you (in the scene). Taste the taste in your mouth. Be there. Be there fully. Then gently, respectfully, remind yourself that you are that person in potential, and with a smooth act of will draw that person in the scene back, as it were, into your present reality and into your body here until they fill you entirely. And now you're that person and that person is you and the reality of that person will manifest in the midst of your reality here.

You have just melded potential reality (the future) with the present. This will bear actual results. Be ready. However, also be aware that performing such an operation – drawing an entire universe into actuality – is a huge feat requiring immense amounts of energy, so take a rest now.

In a state of pure repose, let your mind swim in the picture of what it is you wish to manifest next in your life. Penetrate the picture until you feel you're already in it, living it, loving it and riding it for all it's worth. Then consider the generative force informing its possibility, the pre-atomic substance that is even now giving life to it and will give it its form when the time comes, and allow yourself to feel gratitude towards that force for the picture, as if it's already been brought fully into manifestation. Think, say and feel, 'Thank you.' For while the generative force is the same generative force informing you now as you sit, stand, lie or crouch down reading this, and so is essentially you, and thinking, saying and feeling 'Thank you' is as silly as your hand thanking your arm, the state of gratitude for the materialization of the picture, as if it's already fact, elicits a state of grace. And if this state is intense enough, it will bring you face to face with the generative force, as if it's sitting as an entity in its own right before you right now.

So, rather than wasting energy worrying whether the picture will materialize or not, feel gratitude for its materialization now. This will cause your psychomagnetic field to vibrate at the same frequency as the reality you're bringing into manifest state and is a crucial step in the process.

It requires a willingness to suspend the objections of your rational mind. It requires faith and courage and it requires imagination. But the energy required to feel gratitude for something that hasn't happened yet is far less than the energy spent worrying about whether it will actually manifest or not, and the state of grace it engenders will in any case re-energize you here and now.

At the same time, the instant sensation of communion gratitude triggers will remind you the fruits of your visualization are not the goal. The goal is to know and feel your connection with the generative force, the Tao. In knowing that, you are complete and, in a state of completion, all else will be added to you.

I could keep on trying to sell you gratitude but I guess you'll either buy it or you won't, so I'll just leave it by saying be grateful for what you're about to receive as it will speed things up. Worrying about it will just slow things down. Be grateful.

PURE spirit

Your rational mind will not get this. Use it just to understand the words. Your pure self will get it if you don't get in the way. Getting this will transform your life.

Sit quietly.

Let your weight sink.

Elongate your spine by pushing your neck back a bit and tucking your sacrum under to keep you from crumpling.

Become aware of the ground beneath you, not just directly beneath you but all the way out to the horizons. Tune in to the immense power of it, as it hurtles with you on it around the sun at 66,000 miles an hour, while spinning on its axis at 1,000 miles per hour.

Feel it rushing up along the rear of your spine to your heart (the middle of the chest region).

It's an exhilarating sensation. Settle into it and don't be afraid to enjoy it.

More or less simultaneously, become aware of the heavens above you – the immensity of space in all directions and the immense power contained in it.

Let it rush down through your posterior fontanels (joints in the skull at the crown of the head), down the rear wall of the skull, under the center of your brain and along the front of your spine to the level of your thymus gland (in the center of the top of your chest).

Feel the two energies: the energy of earth and the energy of heaven, wanting to meet in the upper chest but not quite making it. Tune into the tension that causes between the two, which comprises a third energy.

With a gentle act of will, plunge that third energy down along the front of your spine until it settles below your navel.

In this dynamic state of stillness, you will feel your center (the region just below the navel) as the center of the universe.

Allow the you that is experiencing this to be without bounds. Let it be as big as the entire universe, with the energy produced by the tension of heaven and earth meeting and being plunged down below your navel at the center of all existence.

This universal entity is pure spirit.

This is the state from which you manifest your reality.

And in this state you don't care about manifesting reality because you are complete. In completion, all else is added to you.

Do this every day at least once.

Sometimes it will happen for you in a spectacular way and the doors of hyper-reality will open widely and undeniably. Sometimes nothing will appear to happen. And that's the point of practicing it every day. By and by, the incidence of bona fide connection will increase and eventually you'll be living every moment with it going on, at which point you can be said to have reached a state of mastery.

PURE mastery

Being at the center of the universe in a state of alert relaxation, fully in command of the breath and of the moment, as the air comes in and goes out, with your awareness organized in the center of your brain, your spine lengthened, your heart soft, your weight sinking, the earth rushing up through you, the heavens rushing down through you, the energy they produce in their endeavor to meet in your upper chest plunged down below the level of your navel and your spirit as large as the entire universe, while also in the midst of the everyday with its myriad distractions vying for your total attention but not getting it because you're held fast in hyper-reality – that's pure mastery.

And it will come and go. And come again.

That's the nature of mastery.

You will gradually settle into it because it feels better than the alternative but it takes a long time to recognize that, as well as which, occasionally, the pull of external distraction is just too strong to resist and you find yourself lost in following one desire or another.

And you don't punish yourself for it when you spot it happening.

You simply note it and gently draw yourself back into the center zone. You use your breath and adjust your body, plunge the chi of heaven and earth down, know yourself as spirit again and carry on as you were.

No one holds it steady all the time. Someone with more practice than you may give the appearance of being steady in the hyper-reality all the time but they're not. It's all relative. For the advanced master, there are still moments of being in it and being out of it, still moments of doubting the manifestation process, still moments of being drawn away from center by desire for this or that. It just appears that they're holding steady because even at their most distracted, they're still way more centered in the zone than you at your most centered moments.

It's all relative. Indeed, you may be that very master reading this for want of anything better to do. Perhaps you've picked it up at someone's house, while waiting for them to get out of the shower or whatever. And it doesn't matter.

That's why you have to practice every day. The more you do that, the more steady you appear.

Not that appearance is all that relevant in this instant. In fact, it means nothing at all. Mastery is all about what occurs within. By the same token, the more you're mastering yourself, hence the less you're being mastered by externals, the more beautiful you look. It's not that your actual features change shape but the brightness streaming from your eyes and the relative lack of tension in your facial muscles throw your facial set into the best light possible. When you've accepted the state of pure mastery, the state of being purely you, it makes you look better, it makes you shine.

And as I said, it's irrelevant anyway.

Mastery is merely something others see in you.

A true master never considers themselves to be so. They may call themselves one, by way of job description, but they know that no matter how much you master, there's always far more left to master.

PURE acceptance – part two

Pure mastery is only a hair's-breadth distance from pure acceptance and it is worth making the distinction. Mastery is the ability to ride the swing between flipping in and flipping out with maximum relaxation and internal collectedness, regardless of external conditions and circumstances. Acceptance of what is, is a requisite to attaining that state.

Accepting what is does not preclude wishing to improve on it. Accepting does not mean lying down in submission. It means desisting from fighting with reality and wishing it were other than it is at this precise moment. Begin by wishing it to be precisely as it is right now. Be grateful for it. Acknowledge full responsibility for having created it as it is right now. Recall that it is how it is right now because of the stories you were previously telling yourself about the way it is. Relax into it being the way it is.

Relax into being the way you are with it, especially if you're in the flipped-out phase. Relax into being the way you are with it if you're in the flipped-in phase too – but that's easier, so needs less reminding.

Accept yourself right now and accept the reality you've created. From this state of acceptance, you are now free to visualize it changing into something you fancy you'll like even more, something even bigger and more splendid.

Relax your body. Slow down your breath.

Consider how you'd like things to develop in all aspects of your life now. Visualize how you want it to be. Feel yourself to be there, already experiencing it, enjoying it, smelling it, touching it, hearing it, tasting it, watching it, living it and loving it. Feel the smile on your face because of it. Be grateful for it. Accept it. In the same way you can accept things as they are now, both the shade and the light of it, accept the way it is in the vision-version as if it's already happening – with gratitude.

Sit, stand or lie with your arms wide open in a welcome posture, in a gesture of graciously receiving the substance of everything that's about to manifest itself for you. Receive it all with grace. Because, until you do, it can't come to you.

Meanwhile, desist from being so caught up in the idea of making things (or people) come to you that you overlook the nub of the real reward: being who you really are – the pure you, who is complete and lacks nothing.

Take stock of what you're feeling just now – all of it – the pain, the joy, the fear, the excitement, the doubt, the courage, the confusion, the clarity, the blame, the acceptance, the loathing, the love – all of it – hold it all; breathe with it, be with it. Feel your spine lengthening, your shoulders broadening, your body relaxing, your chest softening, your weight sinking, your mind gathering itself in the center brain, and be with it. This is the pure you. Keep breathing through all the loathing and the love, through all the agony and the ecstasy. Focus on the center of your upper chest, where your thymus is situated, and gently raise your breastbone to meet your point of focus. Feel your dignity – your uprightness – and know that no matter what's going on in your mind just now, no matter how much of a hard time you're feeling inclined to give yourself on account of what you perceive as ugliness in your soul, what you are is beautiful and by attuning yourself to that beauty at your core, you will manifest beauty in your life – and it will come to you in myriad forms from all corners, in the appropriate style for you to be lifted up to the next level, bearing in mind that all levels are merely relative to where you're looking from.

PURE service

The point of manifesting pure beauty in your life is to make your life beautiful for everyone to enjoy. The point of manifesting the reality you want is to be of greater and greater service to others. By being of service to others, the world rewards you by being of service to you. This is intrinsic to the mechanism of manifesting the reality you want.

When asking the Tao for guidance about what to do, where to go, whom to do whatever you do with and so on, let your question be, 'How can I serve best, where can I serve best, whom can I serve best?'

The Tao will always guide you in the way to serve best, where to do, how to do it and with whom to hook up in order to do it. You don't even have to understand the guidance intellectually. Just ask the question and let life happen to show you the way, which it surely will.

Turbulence will inevitably arise at times, often soon after asking for guidance. This is indicative of the blockages formed by your resistance being cleared away. You hang onto people and situations, whom and which you're no longer serving, and whom and which no longer serve you, because even though this is restrictive you feel safe in the familiar. As soon as you ask for guidance of how, where and with whom to be of service next, you are required to release whomever and whatever is holding you back. This doesn't mean you need to change personnel, but it does mean you have to change the story you're telling yourself about them in order to allow them space to change around you and to give you the space to change. And that will meet with your resistance and therefore theirs too – it all works by reflection, like a vast hall of mirrors. The same goes for the situations you have going on. You have to change the story you're telling yourself about them in order that they may change.

This could all be just so many words with lots of whos, hows, whats and wheres, of course. And it's not just that.

By being willing to be in service, you are required, by force of circumstances, to let go of many of the stories you've been telling yourself about yourself, the people in your life and the situations you find yourself in. You have to be willing to tell yourself a different set of stories. For instance, tell yourself the story that everyone in your life is a pure expression of the Tao in form and that every situation you find yourself in is a pure expression of the Tao in formation, and that's how reality will show up to you. It will instantly be plastic and pliable, affording you enough flexibility and latitude to make the shifts required to be of most service.

And it doesn't matter.

All that matters in this respect is that if you choose to ask the Tao how, where and with whom to be of service next, the act of asking works as a trigger to transform your life and place you in the flow of the Tao. And that flow will lead you into hyper-reality, whence you are able to manifest the reality you want on the earth-plane in real time. It's not a question of whether it's right or wrong, true or false. It's simply down to doing it and watching how it transforms your experience of being alive here on the planet.

And don't limit your idea of service to the obvious. The way you serve is expressed through whatever you do as you go about the everyday business of being purely you. It could be as simple as inadvertently presenting the image of someone in command of themselves while standing in line waiting to pay at the supermarket, thereby just happening to provide a perfect role model image in that guise for a child whose curious gaze lands on you and whose life suddenly takes on a specific direction as a result. You just never know what effect your presence has on others, even when you're not actively trying to contribute something.

The Tao takes care of the details and exact manner of how your service will be expressed. You don't have to think about it much. Simply being willing to be of service will set in motion the perfect chain of events to facilitate you offering of your unique gift of self through spontaneous moments of pure being. Of course, it helps to have some sort of form through which to express service, such as playing music, writing, dancing, healing, teaching or nursing, as that will focus the effect of service. But even then your real service consists in merely being purely you and through that channeling the force of hyper-reality, the chi, for everyone's benefit.

PURE speed

Service is but a hair's-breadth from surrender and the distinction is worth making.

Surrender to the flow of the Tao is prerequisite for entering hyper-reality. Being willing to be of service, willing to dedicate yourself to service in whichever form that takes, is like putting your hand on the rudder and steering yourself through the rapids.

As I say, the planet is moving at 66,000 miles an hour around the sun as you read this. Consider that speed for a moment. If you were hovering in space far enough away to watch it go by, you'd be impressed by the speed it shot past you.

Yet you find yourself wanting to rush.

You feel an urgency about getting it right before you die.

And that's stupid.

You know it is. I know it is. Everyone knows it is. But rushing to get it right before we die is part of a stupid story we tell ourselves. When you die you won't care how right or wrong you got it by the time you draw that last breath. You really won't. It doesn't matter what happens after you drop your body, if anything at all. You really won't care how right or wrong you had it by the time you draw that last breath. If you'll know anything at all, you'll know that that didn't matter.

Manifesting the reality you want is just something you do to pass the time, because it's better, and more fun all round, than manifesting a reality you don't want. It's that simple. And it doesn't matter.

Knowing this – because you do know it – and choosing to let knowing this inform you with the wisdom you already have but are often in denial of, you stop rushing so much and let the planet do the rushing for you, something it does far more effectively than you, however fast you travel.

By stopping the internal rush and allowing yourself to stop and be here instead, you reach pure speed. By desisting from running interference on the process of manifestation with fearful impatient thoughts based on the erroneous notion that all loose ends must be tied up before departing the earth plane, you allow it to unfold, unfettered, in true elegance.

Tune into the pure speed of now and you are able to manifest what you want instantly, and you don't care because you're satisfied just being here in pure speed.

To boost the activation of this ability, lower your eyelids almost all the way, allowing just a thin slither of light to peep through at the bottom (after reading this first). Draw yourself back into

142

the center of your brain and from there gaze with focused intent up to a point where the hairline should be in the center of the upper forehead and keep gazing until you feel your consciousness pierce the bone and shoot off in a powerful laser-like stream into infinity. The ancient Taoists accredited this practice with giving you power to control your own destiny (whatever that means). The effect in real time is to give you power to manifest what you want instantaneously.

This game has to be balanced with the awareness that you already have exactly what you want and are manifesting it instantly at this very moment. Look around and within you. This is what you want. And you may want to change it.

Having spent a few minutes focusing through the upper forehead, spend time projecting an image of you enjoying having manifested the reality you want as if it's already come to pass, feeling the way you imagine you'll feel then, smiling the way you imagine you'll be smiling. And whatever it takes to facilitate that state on every level will be set into manifestation. It already is because you've been thinking about it and the more focused your thought, the more powerful and surprising the effect will be.

I don't know how it works.

I've never met anyone who does.

I don't know where the Taoists learned it from.

And it doesn't matter.

It works. If you use it, you benefit, and that's all there is to it.

PURE shock

From the moment you drew your first breath you have been in a state of shock.

And you've been dealing with it more or less effectively ever since, so effectively at times that you hardly realize you are in shock any more. And it's all relative.

When you realize it's you who have manifested reality exactly as it is just now, including all the aspects you perceive as giving you grief, specifically in terms of your relationships with others, you are shocked. When you manifest what you're wishing to manifest next, you will be in a state of shock.

This is because by the very nature of the story you've told yourself about reality – being apparently unable to access hyper- reality at will and therefore perceiving there to be a veil across that dimension occluding it from your moment-to-moment experience – you fool yourself into believing you don't know reality is constantly shaping itself to reflect your inner landscape. You are therefore surprised by how things turn out. And it's a good game. It keeps you constantly amused, if not bemused.

On top of which, surprises are great fun. They lend the theatre of your life dynamism and keep you awake and alert.

What's more, you can refine the game by determining that the surprises you receive are magnificent and beautiful, simply by stating to the universe, the Tao, your pure self, that you're choosing that: 'I'm choosing a run of magnificent, beautiful surprises now.' Say that sincerely, then sit back and watch, and before you know it, you'll receive just that. I can't say how this will look, as it's a surprise. That's the point.

These surprises will add to your state of shock about being on the planet in a pleasant way, somehow cancelling out the colder aspect of the state of shock by reminding you that you always have the option to be proactive and if you relax and breathe slowly, you'll enjoy it far more.

Knowing you're in shock explains a lot of things: your angst, the tendency to hold your breath all the time for no reason, your fear of other people, your fear of the environment, your fear of change, your fear of ageing, your fear of failure and your fear of death. You are raw with shock. It's just that you've learned to mask it from yourself and others and they've learned to mask it from themselves and you. We're all pretending not to be in shock. That's why we enjoy art that shocks – it reminds us of what's actually going on behind the pretense, and that's strangely comforting.

Accepting the state of shock purifies it, turns it into pure shock. When you're in a state of pure shock, you are here – you're not pretending and can enter hyper-reality.

Relaxing with the shock gives you command of yourself.

Attracting magnificent, beautiful surprises is a game you play with the state of shock. It's something else to keep you amused or bemused – and it doesn't matter which.

If it resonates with you for a moment and in that moment you feel comfortable in shock and are thus able to set about manifesting something new, it has value; if not, nothing is lost. You can carry on pretending.

PURE intensity

That's the addiction – intensity. You love it. It's why you create reality to impact on your psycho-emotional state the way it does. It's why you create all the drama you do – for the intensity. You do it to remind yourself viscerally that you're alive.

Accepting that, desisting from resisting it, you breathe out with a full exhalation and relax into your body. You're here. You're alive. You're powerful. And you're using it to create intensity.

Where are you feeling it? Check your belly and chest. That's where you collect it.

Soften your belly, soften your chest and feel it disperse around your body.

Notice you feel even more present, even more alive, even more powerful now.

Grasping the intensity and holding it fast in your belly are variously enjoyable and horrible and they're an addiction – a way of locking yourself habitually into a pattern that fundamentally blocks your power from manifesting what you want.

Like any addiction or habit, they're an avoidance mechanism. You're avoiding taking responsibility for manifesting what you want. You're avoiding letting go and allowing life to manifest the changes you want. Because you're scared. You're afraid to let go. That's normal. We're all afraid to let go. That's why we fear death – it's the final letting go.

And it gets easier and easier if you simply locate where you're gripping on in your body and stop it. As soon as you stop gripping, the hitherto trapped energy disperses and circulates, carrying away the psychic debris and introducing fresh potential. Every time you let go, it clears your slate to make way for the new. It's not dissimilar to going to confession and being absolved, except without the rigmarole.

You simply let go and come into the present moment pure.

The pure intensity of what you're feeling in your belly is your lever, your device for accessing what needs to be let go of.

It's a fine thing.

And you must regularly release it and let it flow, otherwise you're blocking whatever it is you wish to manifest.

Hanging in a harness high over a river in the light of a waxing moon, my hands gripped hard on the railing on the side of the disused railway viaduct from which I was about to abseil. It took me a relatively long time to let go. I couldn't see myself doing it. My hands were locked. Then I saw myself doing it in

149

spite of my rational mind and its grip on my autonomous nervous system, and then I was doing it – falling free into open air. It was blissful. That's how it is when you let go. At first you can't imagine letting go of the intensity. Then you visualize it. Then, in spite of the grip your rational mind has on your autonomous system, you let go. And it's blissful.

Only by letting go into the bliss like this can you clear the space for life to manifest the next act in the play for you.

Otherwise all you're getting is reruns. And that's fine. Sometimes there's nothing as comforting as lying in bed all day, watching reruns on TV.

But eventually it gets really boring.

So here we are about to manifest something new.

We're honor-bound to the cause of human evolution to do so.

Recall the psychic loop, running up the rear of your spine and down the front of your spine. Exhale, let go of the intensity in your belly and chest and send your entire perception of reality down the front to shoot out through your perineum between your legs, thus purifying yourself of attachments to everything that has been till now. Inhale and draw the essence of the new reality you want in through your coccyx and up the rear, refining it and strengthening its life-affirming properties as it climbs to the crown of your head and radiates from there to all parts of you, thus setting up an internal resonance with what's about to manifest externally. Repeat this nine times for good measure. At around seven, insert an image of you feeling purely magnificent because all the prerequisite conditions to facilitate your perfect happiness have been met, as you inhale and your perception of reality shoots up the rear of your spine, and then as it goes over the top of your brain and shoots down the front, on exhalation, say thank you, as if it's already come to pass. And before you know it, provided you managed to keep your attention on the text there and didn't let your mind wander off, it will have come to pass and you'll be saying thank you for that too.

PURE Action

Meanwhile, back here in the midst of the pretense and illusion of the everyday – the theatrical devices you use to hide the truth from yourself at every turn and thus make the game more complex and seemingly more interesting – there are actions you can take, pure moves you can make, that place you beyond the pretense and illusion and so act as magic wands, living metaphors, to open the invisible door to the pure simplicity of hyper-reality, whereby as if by magic, all your actions thenceforth become pure. Over the eons, these have been organized into systems. One of the more famous of these is Tai Chi, meaning, literally, the supreme ultimate state, or hyper-reality.

And though I can't teach you it in a book, here's some easy-to-assimilate 'sitting Tai Chi', to give you a tangible sensation of the chi, and the power of the universe it generates, thereby providing a living metaphor for pure action. Performing pure action in ritualistic context by way of setting up a living metaphor, over time, you purify all your other actions with the chi you generate. As well as which, when the chi flows, your intention to manifest something is amplified by the power of the chi that's flowing.

When you actively project an image of what you want to manifest into the chi generated between your hands, it acts in an alchemical way and infuses whatever you're about to manifest with more power. I don't know how this works but it does. As well as which, it feels good. Plus, it is helpful for your vitality levels and is a perfectly viable way to pass the time when otherwise sitting around twiddling your thumbs, being consumed by desire for something you haven't got or generally letting yourself be up-ended by trapped intensity.

Sit comfortably.

Let all your troubles float away on the out-breath.

Let the breath settle into a slow, steady pattern.

Elongate your spine – push your neck back slightly and tuck your sacrum under a bit to give it the most length. Drop your shoulders. Relax your body. Let your arms go heavy. Draw your consciousness back into the center of your brain. Raise your breastbone a touch and soften it. Soften your face. Smile with your eyes.

Bend your elbows to round your arms.

Slowly raise your arms, palms facing upwards, to the level of your navel.

Imagine a fine china plate suspended from above at that level.

Slowly trace the rim of the base of the plate with your fingertips in a circular motion 18 times anticlockwise and 18 times clockwise. Let your fingertips be sensitive and pay attention to the inside of your carpal tunnels (inside your wrists), where you'll feel the chi flowing through after a while, as you will feel it quite tangibly forming a grapefruit-sized electromagnetic ball in your hands.

When you've completed, keep the hands steady, holding the ball in motion.

From the center of your brain, focus on the point in the mid-front hairline on the upper forehead, which when activated puts you in command of your own destiny. Project an image of yourself in the state of already having achieved whatever outcome you intend to manifest in your life next up onto that point. Slowly incline your head forward until your forehead is hanging over the ball of chi in your hands and let the vision projected onto the inside of your upper forehead drip down into the ball.

Now, let the sensation of vision-impregnated chi spread up the inside of your arms into your chest, down below your navel and thence to all parts of you, so that (with practice), you feel your entire body reverberate with the vision and the energy informing it.

Lift your head upright and rest your arms in your lap for a moment.

Repeat the set of movements with the palms facing down, imagining tracing the inside rim of the plate. When you've done, held the hands steady, inclined your head and allowed the vision to drip into the ball, feel the chi spread up the outside of your arms, across your shoulder blades, into your heart (from behind), down to your navel and thence to all parts of you to reverberate, as before.

Lift your head upright and rest your arms again.

Take a bit of notice of how you're feeling. Check for any build-up of intensity in your belly and chest and if you find any, let it go.

Breathe freely.

Visualize a miniature, six-inch-diameter, soldier-style brass-band bass drum strapped to your front.

Slowly trace its rim, using your fingertips, 18 times going from the back under the bottom, up the front and back over the top towards you, ready to start again. Then reverse it for 18 repetitions.

When complete, hold your hands steady with the ball of chi in motion, incline your forehead, let the vision drip into the ball, then let the vision-invested chi spread up the insides and outsides of the arms, to your chest and across your shoulder blades, into your heart from front and rear and then down below your navel to spread to all parts of you.

Focus on the psychic loop now.

Breathe in up the rear and out down the front, allowing the vision-invested energy reverberating in your body to gather itself and start circulating in the loop along with the breath. As it rises in the rear of the spine, feel it becoming progressively refined. As it drops back down the front, feel it becoming progressively purified.

Which is a lot to take in and it's worth it.

PURE Beauty

Rest your mind.

Rest your body.

Repeat nine times, 'I am beautiful in every way and am becoming more beautiful every time I say I'm beautiful.'

Then repeat nine times, 'My life is beautiful in every way and is becoming more beautiful every time I say my life is beautiful'.

It makes you feel beautiful.

Which is when you start expressing pure beauty.

There is no question you've done some ugly things, have said some ugly words, have entertained some ugly thoughts and even pulled a few ugly faces in your time. It's inevitable. Even for saints. And you're probably not one. Relax. Ugliness is essential to the tapestry.

You can't have pure beauty without it.

It's requisite for contrast.

So thank the ugliness you perceive about yourself. Recognize that this is merely perceptual, and not factual, in any case. Appreciate the contrast it provides and having duly honored it, now focus instead on what's beautiful about you.

Are you drawing a blank?

Is your self-destructive tendency telling you there's nothing beautiful about you?

It's normal.

Override it, if so, by listing such aspects as your smile when you're immersed in joy, in love, in amazement, in gratitude, in courage, in vulnerability, in humility, in relief, in satisfaction, in triumph, in ecstasy, in abundance, or in all of them. Go on to list all the times you've shared that smile with others; all the times you've shared your joy, love, amazement, gratitude, courage, vulnerability, humility, relief, satisfaction, triumph, ecstasy, abundance, or all of them. Go on to list how you've kept going along the path, always willing to feel and share who you are.

That's beautiful.

And that beauty shines in your eyes.

Having a relatively symmetrical-looking set of well-toned features to frame it nicely helps too.

To optimize the symmetry and tone of your facial features, stretch and elongate your face as stretched and long as it will go by drawing your upper lip downwards and looking up simultaneously, allowing that to break into a smile once it reaches full extension. Repeat this 18 times.

Draw your chin downwards with mouth closed and contract (raise) your forehead muscles simultaneously 18 times.

Stick your tongue out and look upwards with eyes wide open and release to normal 18 times.

With mouth closed, revolve your chin like a camel chewing in a circular motion 18 times one way, 18 times the other.

Finally, revolve the tip of your tongue around the inside of your gums 18 times one way, 18 times the other. This will work the muscles at the root of your tongue.

Now place a palm on each cheek and rub gently in circles upwards to the temples, then draw the palms lightly down either side of your nose and over your chin, and push back up the sides of the cheeks and temples, down over the cheeks again and so on 18 times.

You'll feel a magnificent sensation of increased blood and energy circulation throughout your face as a result.

Stop, rest and allow your face to relax completely – let all trace of expression slide right off it and feel your entire skull relax.

Wait about three minutes for things to settle then go and look in the mirror.

You'll notice a difference. Your face will look more vital, your skin tone will look healthier and more robust, your facial muscles will be more toned and your eyes will be shining more brightly. Repeat this every day and within no more than 30 days you'll notice your features becoming more symmetrical-looking.

You can pretend it doesn't matter to you but it does.

Having confidence in your face helps you feel more relaxed when you are dealing with other people. As well as which, having a relaxed, balanced face makes others feel better when they are looking at you, which makes them respond to you in person more positively, which in turn increases your confidence, which in turn increases the possibility for manifesting opportunities. Allowing the light of your inner beauty to shine through your eyes more brightly helps light up your interactions with others. The sparkle is infectious.

And there's more to it than that. For if as well as sharing your beauty with others, you wish to draw beauty into your life – beautiful people, beautiful places, beautiful scenes, beautiful objects and beautiful feelings – all you have to do is set up a beauty-resonance within and that will magnetize beauty to you as a pre-atomic ubiquitous essence, expressed in all the people, places, scenes, objects and feelings that make their way into your field of perception.

This actually comprises a refocusing trick, wherein rather than focus on the ugliness, you tune into the hidden beauty at the core of each phenomenon, the Tao informing it with its unique purity and by doing so cause that beauty to ignite and express itself through whatever or whoever is going on around you. Simultaneously hold fast to the beauty as it expresses itself through you. It's a trick and a discipline and not only does it increase the beauty in your own life, it generates more beauty for everyone to enjoy.

Pure beauty is a feeling, a sensation that ripples gently through your chest, causing a quiver. It feels better than ugliness, which gives rise to contraction of the muscles and a general closing-down of the energy field. That's why it's a relatively easy discipline to adopt.

You can try getting high on ugliness but it will ultimately only bring you down. Once you stop fighting it, beauty is a far more elevating substance and smoother and easier to channel once you get used to it.

Walk around saying (to yourself), 'I am beautiful,' for a day and see what a startling effect it has on you and those around you.

PURE vanity

What tends to block the flowering this promises is the fear of losing yourself in vanity.

When you are so obsessed with perpetuating the myth of who you imagine yourself to be, you forget to see the innate beauty of those around you. When you are so concerned with being seen to behave in what you consider to be the expected or appropriate fashion, when you are so fixated on being right about everything, when you are so invested in your future plans and agendas, and when you are so focused on your physical appearance that you forget you are merely a living expression of the cosmos, a humble yet unique flower in the Tao's garden, here to make the world more beautiful by letting shine your particular inner light, these times are when you block the flowering available to you in any one moment – you block the power of beauty that wants to flow from you towards others and vice versa.

Vanity is a distancing device – a way of distancing yourself from the muck and filth of life and death – a way of (vainly) attempting to become immortal.

And there's nothing wrong with that, providing you enjoy the pretense of holding yourself apart from the natural flow in a state of illusory isolation.

In truth, you cannot be apart. There is nowhere in the universe that this is possible, for at the deeper, invisible level, you are intrinsically connected to all that exists, has ever existed and will ever exist.

On the surface of things, you can hold yourself apart and that's where you'll hold yourself: on the surface. But beneath that, in the layers of self that feed you by communing with the generative force of existence as you work, rest and play in the world of the world, you are 100 per cent aware of your connectedness.

This produces conflict in the soul, which can only be resolved by desisting from taking yourself seriously.

But don't be hard on yourself. The whole world runs on vanity. Above all else, people's greatest concern is to look good. And in terms of the world being living theatre, it merely represents low-level acting. When you're acting at a high level, you're expressing the Tao from the very depths of your being outwards, not just from the surface, and that makes you look good. Not that you care. In fact, you take care not to care, as you know that caring only spoils your flow and that spoils your fun.

It doesn't matter what other people think, or what you think other people think about the way you appear. It's not your looks they're after.

Knowing that, you are free to act with the fullness of yourself, with your pure self and are then free to make yourself look as pretty as you like, because you're no longer held to ransom by it. That's when your vanity becomes pure – when you're doing it to make the world look better and not just yourself, when you're doing it for the sake of others, for their visual enjoyment and aesthetic inspiration, rather than to boost your unhealthy attachment to the surface of yourself. For as soon as you realize your presence is experienced by others as merely part of their own play, rather than yours, you've transcended. That's pure vanity.

PURE soul

However, what people want, what turns them on and in turn causes them to want to turn you on by bringing you fresh opportunities in one form or another, is something even deeper than that: soul.

We are, of course, now straying into dangerous territory, not simply because soul is a loaded word in the religious context and a fairly indefinable, highly taste-sensitive one in the musical context, but also because the soul operates on a different dimension – beyond the power of the conceptual mind to grasp, for while it is accessible through the mind-body complex by virtue of it serving as a connector between your local and universal selves, its sphere of communicational connectivity and function exists beyond reality as we know it. It exists in hyper-reality, which is why people so love catching a glimpse of it – it connects them to the causative realm in that instant, hence the value of the arts and the poverty of prose when it comes to my vainly attempting to define it.

There is a degree of two-way inter-dimensional communication flow between the soul and the local self, discernible whenever the heart is stirred, say by love, deep suffering, meditation, shamanic methods (including playing, listening to or dancing to quality music), religious moments, moments of dread, or certain drug-or alcohol-induced altered states. But until the soul is actively accessed, most of it occurs at the psycho-autonomic level, without your knowing about it.

What happens once you access it, is your whole dialogue with the Tao shifts up a level to a higher dimension. It's not that you bring the Tao down to your level, trapping it in the limited myth of who you imagine yourself to be. By accessing your soul, you know yourself as the Tao, not the local, stepped-down illusory version.

So the context of the soul is different to the context of the everyday – it operates on a different set of values.

Once you access your soul, you irreversibly transform the context of your existence and this in turn transforms the content and hence value of your life.

Whether you like the effects of this or not, is again a matter of taste and the catch is, it's a one-way journey.

Your soul has a structure approximately co-spatial with the upper part of the physical body. The references I'm giving here are inadequate but go with it and it can lead you somewhere you want to go, even if you don't know it yet.

Visualize an inverted triangle, its lowest point behind your thymus gland in the center of your upper chest, its flat topside a few feet above your head and sticking out to the sides a few feet. This inverted triangle shape is actually soft and curvy and is textured somewhat like a grossly oversized upside-down seashell that extends upwards and diagonally backwards from the thymus region, under the center of your brain, exiting approximately through the occipital ridge at the rear of the skull and extending way up above you.

It serves as a highly sensitive data-receiving dish, both for information transmitted from the core of hyper-reality and for information transmitted by the souls of those around you, mostly without their knowing.

So, while still in the state of not yet having accessed it, you are not actually receiving others, only your version of them – you are not getting the fullness of the gift others bring you because you're filtering your interaction with them through the story you're telling yourself about them at the time. However, once you access your soul, you find yourself receiving the other fully at the soul level, which radically alters the quality of your interaction with them and vice versa, as well as which you are all at once aware of the information reaching you from the cosmic mind, the pre-atomic consciousness that informs the universe. And you can start doing clever things like accurately predicting the weather simply because your intelligence is now able to discern the subtle pressure changes and make vast calculations that would be beyond the scope of your rational mind to conceive. Not that this in itself would be that interesting, but if you can predict the weather, imagine what you can predict in terms of human affairs.

Hence the word 'psychic', psyche meaning, literally, 'soul'. Once you open the soul you are psychic and can even talk to dead people and vice versa, if the urge takes you that way. You transcend the boundaries of time and space altogether.

Doing so, you are contributing to the human evolutionary thrust.

The way to do it is to lift your breastbone, concentrate on your thymus gland, visualize the inverted triangle-shaped shell extending upwards under the base of the center of your brain, through the lower rear wall of the skull, to high above your head, then be sensitive and expect nothing. You may get a sense of it immediately. You may need to revisit it every day for a few days or weeks, and eventually, providing you keep a thought on it with sufficient frequency, you will get a clear sense of it, as if it were a physical phenomenon.

What will mostly block you is wondering whether you're being daft or insane to be attempting it or even to have believed in it in the first place. And as soon as you get a clear sense of it, you'll stop wondering that.

With a bit of practice, you'll gain great and instant benefit from practicing soul-awareness when you are in the presence of others. You'll find yourself receiving them in a different way altogether and this will transform the experience of communicating with them to one of communing with them.

I wish I could present this in a way that would find favour with your rational mind. I can't. This is the best I can do: to point you in the right direction and give you space to find it for yourself.

However, there's a bit more to it than this. Having received, you are obliged to give as well and it's this function that is governed by the heart, a few inches below the thymus.

You receive with your soul. You give with your heart.

PURE love

The giving is a more local, stepped-down function than the receiving. It happens naturally and spontaneously of itself, as soon as you relax your chest and let it happen.

When you relax your chest and concentrate on making it feel fluid and soft, your heart region automatically transmits love. This love will be picked up by anyone vibrating on a similar frequency.

Pure love isn't necessarily expressed as nice, sweet or even kind. It merely describes a state of remaining open to the world and those around you, specifically in the chest area, so that your natural, innate, human warmth and care can flow freely first to yourself (because if it's not flowing to you, what flows to others will be unreal), and then to those around you, whoever they might be – your partner, a stranger on the street, your friend; whoever – expressed to each in the appropriate way at the time. Not by any particular gesture – you don't need to hug unless you want to – simply by informing your energy field, posture, body language, voice and, of course, scent – and it gets received on a subtle level. You can tell it's happening because the air lights up around you and so do the faces of anyone in your orbit.

It happens of itself, providing you don't stop it.

But you learn to stop it at a young age, usually on account of others around you stopping it with you, usually on account of others around them stopping it with them. And so on, all dating back to the first time someone was hurt because they thought someone else wasn't receiving their love. And that set up a pattern in humans to stop their love flowing, when all along the one thing that makes life good for everyone is having the love flow. If there was an original sin, this was a big aspect of it.

And to some extent you bought into this. At some level you're telling yourself a story that includes a bogus idea that stopping your love flowing is a useful thing to invest your energy in.

Spend a moment relaxing your chest and visualizing warmth flowing freely from there. It's no imaginary phenomenon either. Electromagnetic energy can be measured extending up to 12 feet from your heart.

The heart is about as high as you can go within the body as metaphor, and still remain within the everyday human context of reality. Higher than that and you're into soul territory, where the context is transformed, so learning to play around this level is important. It is in the interface between the human and soul levels that the ultimate alchemy of creating the immortal spirit body is done.

PURE spirit – Part Two

What follows concerns the development of an immortal spirit body. This is the most powerful tool in the book, the orgasm of this body of work, after which it's all down to allowing the spasms to gradually settle as you lie back on the pillows of your mind, assimilate what's happened and choose where you want it to go from here.

Meanwhile, because I haven't died yet (at least not in this body), and am not intending to for a while to come if I can help it, what I'm about to pass on is just hearsay. However, I do have a few close friends who have died along the way, some of whom were engaged in similar alchemical experiments during their own lives and with whom I've been in incontrovertible contact since their passing, who tell me it's not too far off the mark. As well as which, through my tai chi practice I am often in contact with one or more dead Taoist masters, who evidently attained the desired state in their own lives and are thus able to translate themselves directly into the present for my benefit during my practice. I've also noticed that whenever I've been able to connect all the bits in the right way to elicit the sensation of the spirit body, it seems to serve as a powerful catalyst for boosting the process of manifesting whatever I've been wanting to guide into being. And in any case, it feels extremely good on a physical level and even seems useful in terms of preventing fights or dispelling potentially dangerous situations, so I'm fairly convinced it's a viable investment of focus, time and energy. Not that I need to convince you or myself one way or the other. By trying the method you can arrive at your own conclusions. After all, it's all down to the story you're telling yourself and if you're telling yourself one in which having access to an immortal spirit body is a bona fide possibility, then it is. We can only count on reality being subjective.

The ancient Taoists, who either made this stuff up or received it from aliens, were ultimately concerned with developing a structure which exists in potential co-spatial with your physical body, but which is far bigger and operates on a different dimension to it. It includes the soul, which acts as the inter-dimensional connecting agent.

By a relatively simple, yet extremely subtle, so potentially difficult, internal maneuver, you are able to activate the immortal spirit body, or more precisely, activate your consciousness within the dimension your immortal spirit body exists in, and so transform your entire reality at the deepest and highest level.

The main benefit of this is supposedly to not find your consciousness scattered by the event of physical death, leaving you calm, collected and free to continue your evolutionary journey without a blip, which is presumably preferable to the alternative. The secondary benefit of this is a major attenuation of your fear of dying, along with which comes a major increase in your zest for living and for grabbing every opportunity by the horns and riding it for all it's worth.

And it goes like this:

Consider the power of the earth, moving, as previously stated, through space even as we speak at 66,000 miles per hour. Attune yourself to the force of a thrust like that. Imagine over 5,972,000,000,000,000,000,000 tonnes of mountains, rivers, seas, washing machines, cars, people, rabbits and all the rest coming at you through space at 66,000 miles per hour and somehow you manage to trap that force and funnel it up through a small opening between your legs, then feel it rushing up into your chest but stopping at the level of your heart.

Simultaneously, attune yourself to the immensity of space, not just all the air in the atmosphere, weighing in at 14 pounds per square inch, but the imponderable speed the galaxy is moving at and any other reference point you can think of in order to anchor the inconceivable in your mind, and allow the power of all of that to rush in through the upside-down, super-sized, shell-shaped receiving-dish structure of your soul, through the back of your head and down into your upper chest, but no further.

As you feel the power of earth rushing up, feel it rushing up, not just from directly beneath you but from the horizons. Feel the same with the power of 'heaven' rushing down.

Focus on the gap in your upper chest between the downward-rushing heavenly force and the upward-rushing earthly force and on the tension produced by the two attempting to meet and merge. Now, using your will, gently plunge this space of tension downwards until it's sitting below the level of your navel.

If you can hold it steady there for more than 20 seconds or so, you will experience a shift in the very psycho-tectonic plates supporting your entire sense of self. You will feel universal and without limit. If then you are able to draw your mind back into the center of your brain and start revolving light around the loop (up the rear of the spine, over the brain and down the front of the spine, back between the legs, up again and so on), nine times, you will feel as if you're moving that light around the whole universe and somewhere in that process, you'll become aware of yourself as comprising a universally large body made of light, shaped very much like your physical form but more beautiful – and potentially far more terrifying, so don't force it.

Some days you see it instantly, some days you need to sit and concentrate for a while first, other days you don't see it at all. Hence the value of regular practice.

Learning to do this at the drop of a hat means you can switch into it in the midst of daily life and in effect be an instant immortal. This is fundamental to high-level self-defense and will help keep danger and harm away from you. Remember that. Once you can hold the spirit body steady, which is a big once, thus facilitating moments of pure spirit, there is nothing you can't manifest, and the irony is that by the time you can do that you won't care.

But even micro-moments of pure spirit-body awareness will radically transform your reality. That much I can vouch for.

I want to milk this a bit more, give it more noise, but can't think of another thing to say on it except to exhort you to try it out on a regular basis. The only downside I can see about it is that once you have it, you really stop caring about manifesting lesser phenomena such as the accumulation of wealth, so you could say it lessens your ambitions. On the other hand, that won't necessarily lessen your ability to manifest wealth.

PURE wealth

It doesn't matter how enlightened you are, if you say you don't want to manifest wealth you're lying. Even if you're already wealthy beyond measure, you still want to manifest wealth, because wealth is an expression of the life force and life always wants to manifest more of itself. By doing the following you will manifest wealth.

And there is nothing to feel ashamed about.

Wealth is not the root of all evil. Ignorance is.

The more wealth you manifest, the more wealth there will be in circulation for everyone to enjoy. Don't ask me how that works. It's all to do with the law of abundance and you might think that's lazy of me but you don't care, do you? – be honest – you just want to know what to do to manifest the wealth, something you've probably considered the ultimate conjuring trick until now.

However, having reached the stage of glimpsing your immortal self, manifesting wealth is mere child's play.

Start by bearing in mind that every penny you've ever spent or had spent on your behalf represents an investment into the universal bank. Depending on how old you are, what background you hail from and which part of the world you grew up in, you've probably spent out or had spent out on your behalf somewhere in the region of the equivalent of approximately £2 million, give or take a bit. The precise sum is irrelevant. What's important is to get a sense of the immense amount of units of money that have gone into circulation so far on account of you being on the planet.

Now imagine you blessed all that money in retrospect so that its going out into society occurred in an atmosphere of love, so that even the parking fines you have paid were paid with love and good wishes for the recipients, rendering every outgoing penny a happy one. Happy pennies tend to be popular ones. Popular pennies make many friends.

Visualize all the pennies comprising that £2 million or thereabouts moving about society making around 100 friends each, which isn't a lot of friends for a popular penny to make.

Picture them all there now, dotted about the world having fun with all their friends, but all with a vague undefined yearning, a yearning to come home; enjoying themselves but somehow, somewhere deep inside, knowing that they're awaiting that call from home.

Now, using all the tricks learned in this book, expand yourself as best you can into your full, universal size, rise up to all that is beautiful and with sincerity in your heart, address all those pennies. Say, 'Pennies, come home now.' Then visualize every single one of them responding and starting to wing its way back through the veins of the global currency networks towards you, each bringing with them the hundred or so friends they've made while out and about circulating in the world.

So, in case the calculator on your phone isn't handy, this means you are now seeing approximately £200 million wending its way towards you and as your heart starts jumping for joy, before any aspect of your rational mind starts jumping in with boring reasons to spoil the fun, start saying 'Thank you,' as if you can already feel, smell, hear and even taste the money. And as you say 'Thank you,' visualize it starting to pile up all around you, forming a massive heap of money so high you can jump up and down and roll around in it and still not touch the floor. Be there with it.

Feel the sensations in your body. Be purely that person with all that money, feeling gratitude for it. Love it. And return to the everyday state feeling rich. The money will follow shortly from all sorts of unexpected sources. What you don't collect this lifetime will roll over till next lifetime, so don't fret if the full £200 million doesn't all arrive at once. What's for sure is, having performed this exercise with sincerity, you will initiate a flow of enough wealth to supply all your needs from now on. You will reinforce the effect of this by remembering to bless every penny you spend from now on with positive energy and wishes for the wellbeing and abundance of everyone through whose hands that penny will pass – this includes even, and especially, the people who collect the money from your parking fines and taxes.

PURE quality

With the resources fast running out on the planet and us facing potentially the biggest eco-calamity in history, it might seem irresponsible, insensitive, inappropriate and even ignorant to be focusing your attention on manifesting what you want, thereby apparently potentially draining off the resources even faster. But the point of all this isn't to manifest things or situations – things and situations are just the trinkets. The actual reward is the evolutionary jump you've already initiated by focusing on the material in here. This will leave you feeling far more refined in all ways and the more refined you are, the less gross your tastes and desires become. You realize you need less than you thought. You realize the meaning of quality over quantity. You realize you feel better, richer, fuller, more connected, more beautiful and more magnificent when you tread lightly. And so you start to demand less from the environment, you start to demand less external distraction and so your pull on those resources decreases naturally of itself. Multiply the effect of this by the number of people who will read this book and others like it and you start to see and get notable global results.

Attune yourself to the pure quality of your breath and all else will follow. Focus on the life-force carried to you in each inhalation. Appreciate the silken smoothness of the breath. Appreciate the supreme softness of it. Appreciate the sheer magic of its power to keep you alive and let this appreciation spread to all aspects of your existence. Breathe the quality in and breathe the quality back out for everyone else's benefit.

There's no need to sell you the obvious benefits of feeling healthy in respect of enjoying the reality you're manifesting, so I won't patronize you that way.

Let's get straight to it.

PURE health

There is no such thing as 100 per cent health. The body is in a constant state of flux and you, like everyone else, will be in varying states of robust and weak health, according to the time of day, month, year and life, as well as countless other endogenous and exogenous factors. By focusing your visualization powers on what's healthy about you, you cause it to grow, thereby encouraging the force of robust health to take over from the force of weak health. The messages released don't have far to travel. As soon as you've seen the vision, the information is instantly transmitted to your autonomic nervous system and you only need to manifest a 51–49 ratio of robust to weak force to enjoy a state of pure health and be winning the game of staying alive. More than that is a bonus. So you can afford to approach it in a relaxed way.

In fact, relaxing is prerequisite for the force of robust health to grow. Stress causes constriction of the force, thereby weakening it and transforming it into a force of weak health.

Having relaxed a little more, visualize yourself in the space between and behind your eyes from the rear, sitting on 'the healing throne'. Picture a hand lifting a small trap door on the top of your head that you never knew was there and from way up above, a rich, mostly golden, but also containing all the colors of the rainbow, fluid – the elixir of robust health – being poured in slowly like warm olive oil. As if you can see into the body of the projected you, watch the fluid circulate around your brain and your sense organs, bathing and mending every cell, making it new and well, down through your throat, into your thoracic region, circulating around your lungs and heart, then further down into your liver, gall bladder, stomach, pancreas and spleen, then down and back a bit into your kidneys, forwards again into your small intestine, large intestine, bladder, sexual organs, simultaneously moving into your blood vessels, lymph glands, endocrine system, nervous system, bones, soft tissue, and gradually making its way to all parts of you, even to your skin, until you clearly see your entire physical body filled with it, imbuing every cell with robust health.

Now, slowly project yourself forward in through the rear of the projected you and enter fully into that body. Allow yourself to feel fully the great, glowing force of robust health throughout your being. Pay special attention to any specific parts or systems that were hitherto failing you. Incidentally, if your spleen has been removed, the pancreas takes up the juice on its behalf, likewise the liver for the gall bladder, and if you've had a kidney removed, the remaining one takes the extra load.

Once all your cells feel sufficiently bathed, knowing you can and are well-advised to return to this state as often as you feel like it, slowly draw yourself, along with your projected self, back into your body here in the everyday realm again and continue as you were. Tangible results will show up within 24 hours, the strength of which will depend on how focused you were during the visualization. Just as with the visualization for wealth, as well as the visualizations for anything else, you can do this on behalf of someone else with powerful effect. But always begin such a session by seeing it for you, as that will supply you with adequate power and prevent draining your own energy.

PURE protection

Being an immortal spirit you don't need protection, but just for good measure, for the level of self that's bought into the story of you as a finite being, from the center of your brain, project an image of yourself as totally safe and protected from all harm in the midst of a large sphere of blinding white subtle light, extending 12 feet from your spine in all directions (above, below, to the sides, behind and in front), spinning around you, both clockwise and anticlockwise, simultaneously at 186,000 mps, through which only positive, life-enhancing energy can enter, while causing any negative or life-diminishing energy to be spun back to sender.

Slowly draw yourself forward and in through the back of the projected you and feel yourself surrounded by the spinning orb of protective light. Now slowly draw the two of you back into the everyday, here in your body, and allow the orb of light to continue its spin around you.

Reinforce this before leaving home at any time, while out and about, before sleep or whenever you are around people you sense are potentially harmful.

It works.

PURE confusion – Part Two

Regardless of how well-protected and masterful you become in creating realities you want, there will often be this. I'm so confused, for example, I had to write about confusion twice. And that's OK. You can't have pure clarity without it. Or you could, but you wouldn't realize or appreciate it. Confusion is a game you play with yourself by taking many strands of storylines, some imagined, some real, and rolling them together till they form a jumbled, tangled mess of storylines with no space between, thus jamming your thought processes and preventing clarity.

The way through this is not to concentrate on untangling the thoughts but by transcending this level of mind altogether and in the transcendent state simply wiping the mental slate clean and starting again. The system will reset itself simply by closing and restarting the program, in other words.

So don't waste another moment attempting in vain to achieve resolution by pitting one thought-stream against another. Instead, draw the point from which you're bearing witness to existence backwards into the center of your brain. Directly in front of you, in the space between and behind your eyes, project the image of a large, startlingly clear diamond, mysteriously lit from within, turning slowly on its vertical axis in an anticlockwise direction right there in your forebrain, and as it does so it is cooling and cleansing that part of your brain from all thought. After nine or so revolutions, see it turn clockwise for nine revolutions to introduce fresh energy and the essence of clarity to the forebrain. It takes anything from one to 24 hours for this to have full effect.

Try this straight like this or by projecting the visualization onto a slightly future you in the normal way, depending on mood and whim. The main thing is to be able to see it.

In the meantime, allow yourself to relax into the confusion, literally the fused-together state. Breathe slowly, soften your muscles and let yourself be confused. It will pass and inevitably give way to greater clarity, so enjoy it while you can. Accept responsibility for manifesting it initially. Be thankful for it, comprising as it does a sign that you're alive and human. Let yourself revel in being purely confused, trusting it as a necessary part of the gradual, exponential enlightenment process.

PURE spontaneity

Before you know it, you'll be clear as a bell and right as rain, ready to share your clarity with everyone again. For a while, till the next bout. So don't get habituated to clarity.

Shake it up in any case. So much craving for steady and smooth inhibits natural expression. Our whole culture is based on a craving for stability and seamlessness and the price we're paying for that is the potential imminent total destruction of our global life- support system. The same occurs individually. By putting all your energy into making life steady and smooth, you drain off your life- force. Obviously, it's a matter of balancing the two needs: keeping it smooth enough to gain sufficient continuity, while spontaneous enough to allow your life-force to flow.

And don't for a moment take this as an exhortation to turn your whole life upside down, then run down to the nearest shopping mall wearing silly clothes, waving your arms in the air shouting, 'I'm free, I'm free,' sidling up with a semi-crazed smile to strangers, hugging them and telling them you love them, jumping in fountains with evening wear on or anything

191

clichéd like that. You can do all that or versions of it if you feel like it, but the effects I'm thinking of are more discreet, potentially more profound and much farther-reaching in terms of your ongoing existence, something to trigger you beyond wherever you are presently held, in order to open you to whatever run of surprising opportunities lies in wait for you.

Stand up and shake your body, starting at your knees and allowing it to spread everywhere till every cell in your body is shaking, and keep shaking and shaking for as long as you possibly can until you can truly stand it no more, then stop. You'll notice a startling sense of stillness by contrast.

Now, in this state of stillness visualize the power of the Earth rushing up through your feet all the way up to your chest and the power of the sky rushing down through the back of your head into your thymus in the upper chest. As before, feel the tension caused by the two powers wanting to merge and not quite making it. Plunge that tension down into your belly below the navel and hold it there for a moment. That is super-charged life-force. Now allow it to slowly rise up into your chest and as it does, feel it stir your passion. As your passion is stirred, let it cause your arms to slowly rise up to the sides, palms upwards, until forming a T.

Now tune into the pulse of life running through you and start subtly, discreetly, moving your body in an undulating, gyratory

192

manner to the rhythm of the pulse and allowing the motion to extend all the way to your fingertips. By and by, allow the passion in your chest to rise up to the center of your brain and as it does, let your arms extend all the way over your head. Then, suddenly stopping the motion, declare to the universe, yourself and anyone who may be interested, 'I'm free to do anything I choose, I'm free to do anything I choose, I'm free to do anything I choose.' Then settle back into your skin and carry on as you were.

Repeat this simple process, which might last an average of four minutes, each day for three days and significant shifts will occur in your style of operating. You'll find yourself expressing pure spontaneity at the most unexpected moments, and in so doing you'll get to know aspects of yourself you'd never met before. This is one of the main benefits and blessings of engaging in the manifesting process: getting to know fresh aspects of yourself along the way, for it's never the actual achievement that rewards you, it's the expanding awareness of who you really are – the Tao – meeting yourself in hyper-reality.

PURE nonsense

Ichhlackenow potelisoshosh mactulaben po oi po tot. I say this because the rational mind has such a grip on things that to enable the magic of the manifesting process to flow, sometimes you need to loosen its hold, and one of the swiftest methods to do this is taking yourself off somewhere private and talking gibberish for a while. This shouldn't be difficult, as most of what we talk is gibberish anyway, just dressed up in proper language and syntax. All this involves is letting go of that veneer and allowing the unadulterated sound of nonsense to fly from your lips. Indeed, something that never fails to astonish me is how easy it is to induce an entire audience to start talking gibberish aloud, which leads me to believe we're all just bursting to do it and will do it providing someone gives permission. So here it is.

Allow the sounds to come from deep inside. Do not control them with your rational mind. Override inhibition and let whatever nonsense wants to be said to be said. Once you get past that sticking point, it flows of itself. Allow your vocal range to slide where it will, from falsetto to bass and back again.

Explore strange groupings of consonants and vowels and be emotive with it. You can instantly tell how stuck and up their own ass someone is by how freely they're able to let go into this, which is my gentle way of bullying you into it, for surely you don't wish to give the impression of being anal.

Paradoxically, after a ten-minute gibberish session, you'll notice your communication skills using structured language have increased noticeably.

In terms of hygiene on a psycho-emotional level, I'd place this along with voiding your bowels on a daily basis.

And it's equally rewarding with respect to how it leaves you feeling: light and nimble, free of whatever set of serious thoughts were hitherto weighing you down.

From pure nonsense, then, comes pure wisdom.

PURE wisdom – Part Two

You've probably noticed a growing undercurrent in the preceding chapters, an implication that you're still going to be fallible even once you have accessed your soul, your spirit body and all the enlightenment these will bring you; that even with all the most powerful manifesting tools known to humankind, you are still going to mess things up and you may think this is out of place. But it's not.

Of course you are going to mess things up. In fact, the more enlightened and hence powerful you become, the more likely you are to mess things up and the more dramatic your messes will probably be.

Wisdom consists in knowing that being flawless is not only not the point of the game, it's also impossible, and that being flawed is not only intrinsic to the game, it's what makes it worth playing. Indeed, were you flawless, apart from the fact that you wouldn't have incarnated in the first place, you would have no interest in manifesting or not manifesting anything. You would simply be and would have no urge to do anything, which is why it could never be the case. The tension between being and doing provides the necessary friction for personal growth, so even though you aspire to a state of pure being, with all your doings so pure you don't notice it happening, this merely represents a direction rather than an attainable goal. Understanding and accepting this constitutes wisdom. Understanding and accepting you're a fool constitutes wisdom. Understanding and accepting that confusion is inevitable constitutes wisdom. Understanding and accepting that doubt, fear, greed, small-mindedness, nastiness, dishonesty, vanity and all manner of undesirable states are also inevitable from time to time constitutes wisdom. And understanding and accepting that fleeting moments of understanding and accepting that all the preceding is merely a story I'm telling you, and that you're telling yourself, and so is not ultimately true, constitutes pure wisdom. Understanding and accepting that you don't really and never will really understand or accept anything fully, including the keys to manifesting the reality you want, constitutes wisdom.

And when you can read all that and think, 'What?', even while knowing precisely what I mean, even knowing it's possible you totally wasted money on this book to find out something you already knew (that you didn't really know anything), yet also getting that something deeper beyond the scope of the rational mind is being transmitted nonetheless – while also knowing

that could be a cop-out and con likewise, but not really caring –
that constitutes wisdom: pure wisdom.

PURE play

Self-help will eat itself. It must or it would mean it hadn't worked. Eventually everyone is helped and the method becomes redundant. Understanding and accepting that and understanding and accepting that we haven't reached that stage yet constitutes wisdom. Understanding and accepting that none of it matters beyond having provided a pleasant way to pass the time constitutes wisdom. And you probably think I'm playing with you and I am.

I'd be surprised if you weren't enjoying it. Playing is good.

We spend too much time being scared to play.

One of the sickest developments of recent times has been the marketing of play. It's an extension of prostitution that has put a price on everything, including someone's company, rendering there a dearth of pure play, which is sad because pure play is the most powerful way to touch the divine and is actually what everyone is looking for at all times. It's hard to define play.

Losing yourself is the key, as in losing the constructed aspects of your self to reveal the pure you at the core of your being. It's the reason people like to get drunk, stoned and out of it: to lose themselves. Why would we want to? Because carrying around the nonsensical story of who you think you are meant to be is so limiting, so restrictive and so boring, so violent towards the real magic of existence, we need strong anaesthetic to break it down.

But imagine no longer feeling obliged to carry that nonsense around with you. Imagine dropping it on the floor with a thud and saying, 'Enough is enough,' then moving on as light as nature intended you, without pretense, without contrivance. You would then automatically find yourself in a state of play with life. The world would be your playground. Manifesting realities would be the game you played. Messing it up would be your major source of amusement. Getting it right would be your major cause for glee. Understanding both are illusory would be your main source of entertainment. Wondering how to fill the gap previously filled by fighting incessantly with yourself would be your main challenge. And this would be translated into everything you did, not just in your so-called leisure time, for leisure time is part of the story of your life only partly belonging to you. It would translate into your work time, your rest time and even your sleep time as well. You would be playing all the time. Sometimes the game would get a bit dark, as games do. Other times it would be startlingly bright. Neither shade would have major impact on your level of enjoyment.

You would have transcended preferences. You would know that what you were playing with was the Tao and in so knowing would know that in actual fact it wasn't you playing with the Tao but the Tao playing with itself and, in that moment, would find yourself bang at the heart of the cosmic manifestation process, which would probably be a bit much for you to take in so you'd all but instantly flip back out of that enlightened state into the stepped-down human version of self you're more habituated to, like stepping off the mountain peak you'd spent all day climbing to reach because the wind was too powerful and the view too big. And your stepping off the peak would be a source of amusement and enjoyment and you'd probably congratulate yourself at that point for being so wonderful, which is where it would all start going wrong.

PURE arrogance

The distance between pure arrogance and pure vanity is less than a human hair's width, but the distinction is worth making. Pure vanity arises from the delusion that you created yourself from scratch. Pure arrogance arises when even though you know that isn't so, you congratulate yourself on being very clever for playing the game with the Tao well. And it's inevitable. Whenever you experience a run of things going your way, arrogance sets in. It's insidious. It creeps up from behind when you're not watching and infests your communication with others, blinding you to the fact that they too are expressions of the Tao and that really no matter how clever you've been, even had you managed to manifest the greatest life and set of conditions in recorded history, compared to generating an entire universe, your own enterprise is paltry. Arrogance draws your energy upwards and makes you top-heavy, hence easier to knock off balance. An intrinsic part of the game you're playing with the Tao, and vice versa, centers around you withstanding oncoming forces and maintaining your balance, so any time the Tao feels you being top-heavy, it will naturally give you a push that will up end you. And that's fine. Being up ended is fun if you're willing to let go of looking good.

Real power derives from channeling the Tao humbly.

Try this exercise.

Take yourself to a fashionable part of town where lots of people are busily running hither and thither, obsessed with the game of looking good, and walk slowly in their midst by taking extremely small steps of only three inches, as if wearing very tight leg-irons. Do not change this even when people start looking at you strangely, which they inevitably will. Complete at least 30 yards' distance before allowing yourself to walk normally again.

Alternatively, if that sounds too subtle, go to the same area wearing a pair of false ears.

PURE elegance – Part Two

Having visualized an outcome you wish for and followed some or all of the techniques for refining and intensifying the process of setting it into manifestation, you will sometimes, if not often, be beset by trials. This will be on account of blockages within your system, as well as blockages in the world around you, causing major disturbance to the flow of energy required to bring what you want into being. This is not to be feared or resisted. Indeed, the more readily you can accept the trials that befall you with grace, the more swiftly you are able to glimpse and appreciate the pure elegance inherent in the way the scenario unfolds, not in spite of the blockages but because of them.

Blockages are essentially illusory and therein lies the clue to dispelling them. Understand that they don't really exist and are merely theatrical devices there to make the story more exciting and dynamic, understand that at the deepest level you already have everything you want, understand that they only present themselves to afford you a chance to examine how committed you are to manifesting the new reality. Above all, understand that contrary to appearances it's you who have manifested them and the blockages tend to disperse of themselves without too much delay.

The key is to remain focused on the reality you're wishing to manifest rather than on the apparent blockage.

Nonetheless, it will always be helpful to visualize yourself jumping clean over every blockage and to see yourself on the other side looking back, feeling exuberant for having cleared the way. This applies no matter how apparently large or insurmountable the blockage before you – whether it's apparently being caused by someone close to you or someone you don't even know – simply see yourself jumping clean over it and standing on the other side with a smile on your face.

Generally, the bigger the blockage, the bigger the subsequent release. That's where the elegance is: in watching the blockage disperse. But it's hard because you're human and you get impatient and doubtful; you start comparing yourself to others and get beside yourself with confusion. Were you able to remain centered, calm and focused on yourself, rather than holding yourself up for comparison, you'd find it a lot easier. You wouldn't take the trials so personally and would therefore waste far less energy fighting with yourself over them.

Elegance happens of itself whenever given space. Look at the universe. Look at the planet. Look at nature. Look at the oceans. Look at people. It's all pure elegance in motion.

Tuning into the inherent elegance in all phenomena increases the elegance in your soul, which in turn increases the elegance with which things work out for you. Repeat a few times, 'I love this elegance.'

PURE grace

Accept what's happening to you right now with softness in your heart, without questioning the wisdom of it, without questioning the wisdom of the Tao for making it be so, without questioning the wisdom of yourself for having manifested it, with a trusting, loving heart, and you are in a state of grace. Be expectant of full delivery from all pain and deprivation without giving way to believing the doubts in your mind and you are in a state of pure grace. Be happy for and wish well to others who appear to have manifested what they wanted, rather than give way to envy or disdain and you are in a state of pure grace. Be willing to keep your heart open and your love flowing through all the pain and hardship of being you, and you will be in a state of pure grace.

It's in the state of pure grace that things start manifesting for you. Not that that's why you engender it. You can't contrive it. Grace happens of itself when you get too tired to keep fighting with yourself and the world and start allowing it to be as it is because you haven't got the energy to waste doing otherwise any more.

That's why you must learn to welcome the pain of resistance – not through misplaced masochistic tendencies, but because you know it is a prelude to grace.

Grace and gratitude are so close you could almost miss the difference, but the distinction is worth making. Grace is the state that allows gratitude to flower. Once you can start saying thank you for how you find yourself, including all the pain of resistance, the pain of resistance disperses of itself. Once you can be grateful for having manifested whatever mess you perceive before you, the mess instantaneously starts transforming itself into a miracle.

PURE strength

To hold steady through the vicissitudes unleashed by the manifesting process you need strength. Pure strength is a pre-atomic quality and is the same whether channeled through the body or the mind. It's more tangible, hence easier to access through the body, however, and here's a foolproof way of doing it.

Stand with your feet at shoulder width, both feet facing forwards as if you are standing on train tracks, with knees slightly bent, sacrum lightly tucked under, back of neck pushed back a bit. Push your arms behind you, palms facing backwards, arms almost straight. Open and close your fingers 49 times as if grabbing and releasing something. Bring your arms parallel with the sides of the body in a gunslinger's pose and repeat. Raise the arms in front of you to shoulder height, palms facing downwards, and repeat. Turn the palms upwards and repeat. Swing the arms out to the sides, palms facing upwards to form a T, and repeat. Turn the palms to face downwards and repeat. Raise your arms above your head, palms facing forwards and repeat. Finally, bring the arms down in front of the belly as if holding a bowl at navel height and repeat.

You will notice your arms feeling quite paralyzed during the process. Take no notice of this and simply continue, remaining as relaxed as you can throughout, and breathing freely.

When you've completed all the movements, shake your hands gently and release all the accrued tension.

Perform this every day and, within only three days, you'll notice a marked increase in your overall body strength, as well as your mental focusing strength, and will generally find yourself able to exert a far steadier grip on reality. Plus, it will make your hands look nice.

PURE mystery

That's what it is, this game of manifesting reality: pure mystery. For though I confidently assert this and that throughout the book, implying that I know one way or another how it all works, I haven't really got a clue. I'm not ashamed of that. No one has a clue. I can point to the mechanics and say that by following various procedures, certain outcomes can be expected with some degree of certainty, but in actual fact it's all experimental and I haven't a clue what I'm talking about. For instance, you could follow every prescription in this book diligently, get yourself into just the right space, have all the requisite elements in place and then suddenly die tomorrow. I'm not saying you will and sincerely hope you won't, yet it remains a possibility and one I wouldn't know how to explain. In other words, all this, at best, is a game we're playing while we hang around waiting to die and so we must desist at all times from taking any aspect of it too seriously.

I don't mean to undermine myself, you or the material by saying this. On the contrary. I just wish to put it all in clear perspective. There appears something arrogant to me in asserting too boldly what's what about the ineffable mystery of life and I wish to dismantle any tendencies towards that that this book may have elicited so far.

So it's not about judging the information wrong or in any way deficient, nor is it about judging it right or sufficient. Judging it is not what it's about. It's about suspending judgement and humbly following the steps suggested, knowing confidently only that what will follow is a mystery, how it works is a mystery and what it will bring is a mystery

Partly I do this because I know that setting off a process of manifesting a new reality will send such power into the sea of infinite possibility that at first you are severely splattered with the backsplash and can often lose your footing, to the detriment or delay of the ensuing manifestation. And so to preclude that I am wishing to firmly anchor the idea that anything could and probably will happen next and is best welcomed rather than resisted.

If you wish to meld with the mystery more, with every thought you have, word you say or action you take, repeat the question, 'Whatever next?'

PURE luck

Luck is mysterious. Some say you make your own luck. Writing a book like this I could be saying that myself. And though I would have vehemently supported that view in the past, as I've aged and mellowed I've had to concede that there are times when it appears as if some mysterious, ineffable force operates totally beyond our understanding of cause and effect, beyond our understanding of right and wrong, reward and punishment, beyond superstition, beyond praying or being nice to the Tao, beyond building up a storehouse of good deeds done, beyond wearing particular colors, beyond the way we arrange our work or living space according to the precepts of feng shui, beyond whether we avoid walking under ladders and even beyond being clear as a bell in our intention to manifest any particular reality. And this force is luck.

It could be nonsense. It could just be a lazy way of avoiding explaining the complex workings of cause and effect. It could be something that exists only because you write it into the story you're telling yourself about reality. Or it could be an actual phenomenon in its own right.

I don't know and nor does anyone else. I think it would constitute pure arrogance to curtly disclaim it as mere delusion simply to fit in with a particular ethos of being responsible for your own reality. It's a paradox, I know, but then the entirety of existence rests on paradox as a basis.

My inclination is to say it's nonsense. I just can't do so 100 per cent. I don't know how you feel about it. And it doesn't matter. What matters is that if ever you are of the mind that what is happening is as a result of luck, dispense with the besmirching effect of superstition and let it be pure luck: neither good nor bad, just pure – pure, mysterious luck. For in the purity all paradox is dissolved.

PURE luxury

There's nothing intrinsically evil or sinful about luxury. Luxury is an expression of the Tao – the word itself literally means an outpouring or expression of light, and it doesn't have to be a heavy resource drain. Luxury is more about the way you feel in relation to the air you breathe, the sensations in your body, the miracle of your consciousness and about your ability to communicate what you're thinking to others, the joy of relating and the sensual pleasure derived from interacting with all aspects of reality. By attuning yourself to luxury in all you think, say and do, you tend to draw the luxurious towards you, without even thinking about it.

Luxury does not necessarily imply ornate décor or ludicrously priced clothes, exotic food flown from the other side of the planet or even first-class air travel, though it can include all these and more. It is actually a state of being, in which you perceive the luxury in every phenomenon and in your capacity for experiencing every phenomenon, from the humblest to the grandest. It is a state in which you are fully in command of your own timetable, your own life, in which you are no longer making choices based on what you imagine others expect of you, in which you are making choices based solely on what feels right to you in every cell of your body, in which you are able to say what you mean and mean what you say, even when you mean no, in which you are free to come and go as you please, in which you are always equipped with adequate wherewithal to support whichever option you choose from moment to moment, and in which no matter what, you always feel like the king or queen of no matter what.

Luxury is having whatever you want and wanting whatever you have. Attune to it here and now by training your mind and emotions to be in a state of wanting everything you currently have, including the bits you don't like. Meditate on it for a few moments until you can say, with all your heart, on looking around and within you, 'I want all this.'

The need for gold leaf and other trappings of luxury falls away the more at one with pure luxury you become, and simplicity starts to take your fancy progressively more, not that there's any accounting for taste; there are always exceptions to the rule and it's not for me to get involved in that level of your life... however, with resources dwindling it would make sense that the collective consciousness's evolution would take us each towards simplicity now, so don't fight the urge.

Spend a moment visualizing yourself from behind in a state of luxuriating in reality. Note the body language and posture of that person. The clothes. The footwear. The hairstyle. Imagine you can see a faint golden glow around the fingertips of that person, as if they possess the golden touch. Then slowly, gently, move forward into that person until you inhabit their body. Feel what it is to luxuriate in reality. Feel what it is to be surrounded by luxury and slowly draw the two of you back into the present moment. Pure luxury will follow, starting any time now.

PURE terror

You can't avoid it. Occasionally you will be gripped by it and it doesn't matter how spiritually primed you are, nor how much you include being unafraid in your visualizations, there will be times it grips you right deep down from the guts upwards. And it's nothing to be ashamed of. On the contrary. Were you never to feel pure terror, you could not validly claim to have fully incarnated here on the planet. Pure terror is intrinsic to the Tao. If asteroids have consciousness, don't think for a moment they don't feel terror just before crashing into a planet. If galaxies have consciousness, don't think they don't feel it just before being swallowed up in a black hole. Animals feel it just before being eaten alive in the wild. People feel it from the moment they're born. It's just that one of the jobs of the rational mind is to reassure us that at least in the short-term, there is nothing to feel terrorized by, without which function we'd be unable to effectively negotiate our way through a typical day or night. Terror is the heart of all experience and rather than fight or deny it as if it was some shameful disease, far better to embrace it to the extent that you are willingly quaking in your boots, for in

218

the quaking you will know the power of the Tao and in knowing that you have entered hyper-reality and are thence able to reshape reality according to your will – more or less.

Use terror as a catalyst for touching the Tao and thereby doing your magic with.

To refine and channel the force of terror, give your lower back a bit of a massage for a minute or two, using your knuckles to knead in a circular motion either side of your spine at waist level, for this is where fear gets trapped in your body. Use your mind to relax the region and sensitize yourself to the freed-up energy circulating around your body. Breathe slowly and deeply and simply allow yourself to feel the terror spread around you until it is no longer pure terror at all, just pure – purely you.

You will have done yourself a great service.

You need the terror to support the manifesting process, but it can only do this if it is free to be what it is and to circulate freely all about you.

PURE confidence

If you didn't persist in driving yourself half-mad with self-doubt and undermining fearful thoughts at every turn, you would naturally be supremely confident – literally meaning, you would trust yourself. The more you trust yourself, the better you perform on your own behalf in terms of the choices you make. It's the same as with any leader: the more trust in the leader, the better job they do.

Imagine it. Imagine if you didn't constantly undermine yourself with all those negative thoughts about yourself, all that doubt. You would be so much more relaxed about everything, so much more at home in the universe. And the more relaxed and at home you feel here, the more able you are to manifest what you want. It's all down to confidence and you don't actually need to do anything special to develop confidence. You simply have to stop doing what you've been doing almost all your life to get in the way of it.

Confidence is the natural state.

If you could remain with all your muscles fully relaxed, with your breathing flowing freely, with your spine lengthened and your breastbone raised, with your weight sunk below your navel and with your mind drawn back deep into the center of your brain, your heart open at all times, even when feeling pure terror, no matter what was occurring around you – you would be feeling supremely confident. You would be trusting yourself with every choice, not only those that you're about to make but all those that you've ever made. If you could maintain that state consistently, you would never waste another moment doubting the choices you've made, even if they occasionally appear to have landed you in the crapper. You would never again waste a moment doubting the choices you're making as you go along. You would simply know with every bone in your body that every choice you make is the right one for you and that it doesn't matter anyway. That's pure confidence.

Which then naturally extends itself into feeling supremely confident in personal, social and professional situations. You would trust yourself implicitly simply to be you, and that would be good enough. Way good enough. There couldn't be anything better, in fact.

It won't happen, however – and I'm confident in saying that – because you, like me, are addicted to playing games with yourself to make life more challenging, as if it isn't challenging enough as it is. So you beleaguer yourself with undermining thoughts of fear and self-doubt, attacking your self-esteem for any and every reason you can find, the result of which is you've forgotten how to trust yourself and how good it feels when you do.

So, to remedy that, some method acting is required.

Take yourself into the meditation state and lower your eyelids almost all the way.

Gather your consciousness in the center of your brain. Imagine you are someone who has never learned to play the silly game of self-undermining. Gaze deep into the space between and behind your eyes and repeat at least 81 times with feeling, 'I trust myself.'

PURE passion

Without passion, your life is worthless. It may be all neat and tidy, but it will have no real value. Passion is whence caring arises. Without caring, nothing means anything and you are lost. For though everything in existence is changing and has no real intrinsic value in itself, you have to care about things – you have to care about people and you have to care about yourself. You stop yourself feeling passion because you're afraid it will hurt when you inevitably get separated from the object of your caring. But you will actually feel more pain that way because you will never take the value when it is there to be taken. It's far healthier to feel the passion fully and also feel the pain that goes with it.

At the same time, the more evolved you become through the practice of everything in this book, along with whatever other spiritual practice you engage in, the less you take the passion or the pain personally. It still hurts, but whom it hurts you're not so heavily identified with. This enables your core to remain relatively unruffled as you make your way through the meetings and separations of life.

Relax your chest. Feel the passion there. Breathe freely with it. Relax your body. Be with it. And let it inform you henceforth. Otherwise, though you may develop masterful manifesting skills and create the best reality anyone's ever seen, a truly cold fish you'll be and you won't enjoy it, which would be stupid.

PURE comedy

Prepare yourself, for having engaged with this material to this point, you will have already set in motion an irreversible flow of events in your life and what will follow will inevitably be purely comedic. At least, that would be the best way in which to experience it all. Take any aspect of it too seriously, including your death or the death of those you love, including even the end of the world as you know it, and you have already gone way off the point.

Place your fingers under your lower ribs, right hand on the lower right-hand ribs, left hand on the left, and gently prise your ribcage apart an inch or so. Keep breathing and keep prising. Keep your shoulders and elbows relaxed throughout and eventually, when you've had enough, let go all of a sudden and fake a laugh: 'Ha, ha, ha, ha, ha, ha!' etc., until you find yourself laughing spontaneously and keep that going at some level for the rest of your life. If the Tao has any sense at all, it has a sense of humor. When you lose yours, you've lost touch with the Tao, so keep laughing even when it hurts. Especially then.

PURE service – Part Two

Saved till last because it's the most important thing in the book but would be relatively meaningless without the preamble, the following visualization comprises an act of pure service and entails visualizing a world for future generations. Because if this stuff works, there can be nothing more important than to create a reality that facilitates that, unless you're totally self-centered and don't care about the human experiment beyond how it affects you personally, in which case skip this and move straight to the final chapter.

Otherwise, take a moment to settle yourself within your skin. Lengthen your spine, drop your shoulders, raise your breastbone, soften your chest, sink your weight below the level of your navel, breathe slowly and freely and draw your mind back into the center of your brain. From here, project your consciousness along a line stretching out into infinity in the void between and behind your eyes, approximately 100 yards along that line, until it finds itself in a potential future world, a few generations along from now.

As you look around, notice how still it all feels, how peaceful and how harmonious. Note your surprise at that. Notice also how clean and fresh the air smells and feels to breathe. Notice also the lushness of the landscape. Notice also the hum in the air hinting at people working in seamless cooperation with each other. Recognize how this can only have come about through an evolution of consciousness. Notice that the land has neither been inundated by the sea nor poisoned with chemicals. Note how your mind can clearly detect, present everywhere, a higher level of consciousness than anything currently available. Recognize that this could only have come about had there been no devastating wars, no cataclysmic earth-changes, no clamp-down by military-style government on personal freedom and no takeover by tribes of opportunistic gangsters. Make it as Utopian as you possibly can. Prevent your rational mind jumping in with reasons why not. Place a haze of white protective light around the vision, smile, clap your hands and say aloud, 'Let it be so.' Return to now and carry on as you were.

PURE fact – Part Two

You are here.

You are powerful.

And you're not blocking it so much now.

Not nearly so much.

And something amazing is already coming your way.

There's nothing you can do to stop it now.

Relax, surrender, be grateful and receive.

Job done.

Till next time…

Also by Barefoot Doctor:

'The Tao of Sexual Massage' with Jurgen Kolb Gaia Books (1992)

'Barefoot Doctor's Handbook for the Urban Warrior' (1998)
also published as 'Barefoot Doctor's Guide to the Tao: A Spiritual Handbook for the Urban Warrior' (1999)

'Barefoot Doctor's Handbook for Heroes' (1999)

'Barefoot Doctor's Handbook for Modern Lovers' (2000)

'Return of The Urban Warrior' (2001) republished as 'Tao if Internal Alchemy' (2017)

'Instant Enlightenment' (2004) republished a 'This is the Key' (2017)

'Manifesto' (2005) republished as 'Tao of Manifestation' (2017)

'Dear Barefoot: The Wisdom of the Barefoot Doctor' (2005) republished as Taoism for the Mainstream (2017)

'Invincibility Training' (2006)

'The Man Who Drove With His Eyes Closed' (2009) *also published as 'Supercharged Taoist: An Amazing True Story to Inspire You on Your Own Adventure'' (2010)* republished as 'Driving with Your Eyes Closed' (2017)

'Jewels of Enlightenment' Nightingale Conant (2009) (audio)

'The Message' (2012) republished as 'If Moses was a Taoist' (2017)

'Awakening the Laughing Buddha within' (2013) with Joe Hoare

'The Tao of Positive Noise' (2017)

'Superhealing' (2017)

'Self-Love'

'Great Presence'

For all these books and more visit

www.waywardpublications.com

For more on Barefoot Doctor - wisdom, events, and more, go to

www.barefootdoctorglobal.com